T.T.Y.L P.C.O.S

A guide to living with PCOS, without the symptoms

By: Tamara C. Kelley

Dedicated to the two most supportive people I know.

Without my son and my husband none of my dreams would have ever came true.

I thank them for never giving up on me.

Table of Contents

Introduction

To all my beautiful cysters, welcome!

TTYL PCOS originally became a thought back in 2013. I was newly diagnosed and like many others, I was finding helpful information regarding PCOS to be rather scarce. I felt scared and alone with a dysfunctional body. I knew something was wrong with me, I was living it every day. Although I had been experiencing many issues since 2004, it wasn't until I heard those words, "You have PCOS"; that everything became real. It was a very definite and numbing feeling.

Polycystic Ovarian Syndrome affects an estimated 6 million women in the United States alone. That statistic includes mothers, daughters, sisters and friends. One out of every ten women of child bearing age will get it.

As a matter of fact, it's the most common endocrine disorder in women. It is also the most overlooked and misdiagnosed condition. Most women don't know they have PCOS until they begin struggling with infertility and start seeing doctors for help.

The sad truth is PCOS has no cure; however the symptoms can be managed through consistent lifestyle changes. It's all about finding what works best for your situation and your body.

Disclaimer

Please understand, I am not a doctor nor do I claim to be one. None of the lists provided in this book are exhaustive. There are many other treatments that could work for PCOS symptoms that are not included in this book. The contents of this book are intended for women with PCOS. Also note that everyone's body, symptoms or situations are not the same. There for there is no guarantee anything contained herein will be effective for you. Managing PCOS symptoms is a lot of trial and error to find a combination that is best suited for you. The information contained in this book is not intended as medical advice, nor should it be solely relied upon as a substitute for talking with your physician. Always consult a licensed medical professional before beginning or changing any form of treatment.

CHAPTER 1: ABOUT PCOS

History of PCOS

PCOS was first discovered in 1935 by two American gynecologists from Chicago. Irving F. Stein Sr. and Michael L. Leventhal named this condition after themselves, calling it Stein- Leventhal Syndrome. Irving and Michael named it at Michael Reese Hospital.

Ancient medical records indicate that while this condition did not have a name just yet, there were cases many years before it was actually discovered in 1935. Hippocrates (460 BC- 377 BC) mentions the symptoms and says "But those women whose menstruation is less than 3 days or is meager, are robust, with a healthy complexion and a masculine appearance; yet they are not concerned about bearing children nor do they become pregnant." (Diseases of women 1.6) (1)

Soranus of Ephesus (C. 98 – 138 AD) was a Greek obstetrician and gynecologist who was also a chief representative of the Methodist school of medicine. He wrote "[S]ometimes it is also natural not to menstruate at all. It is natural too in persons whose bodies are of a masculine type. We observe that the majority of those not menstruating are rather robust, like mannish and sterile women. (*Gynecology*, Book I. Art. 23 and Book I. Art 29) (2)

Moises Maimonides (1135 – 1204 AD) was a physician. He reported "there are women whose skin is dry and hard, and whose nature resembles the nature of a man. However, if any woman's nature tends to be transformed to the nature of a man, this does not arise from medications, but is caused by heavy menstrual activity." (*Fin Liber Comm. Epidemirum* VI, 8) (3)

PCO vs. PCOS

Pah-lee-SIS-tik-OH-vuh-ree-SIN-drohm

I'm sure you've heard of PCO and wondered the difference between that and PCOS. Is there even a difference? Of course there is! I'll tell you- PCO stands for Polycystic Ovaries. You can have PCO without technically having PCOS. The reason behind that is because PCOS is Polycystic Ovarian Syndrome. The difference between the two being one is a syndrome. To have a syndrome, you would need to have other symptoms in addition to the cysts on your ovaries. A syndrome typically means a group of symptoms such as polycystic ovaries, hirsutism and amenorrhea.

While the symptoms of PCOS are frustrating, there are more reasons than just the inconvenience to get them under control. It's very important to maintain regular appointments with a doctor who understands not only the long term risks associated with PCOS but also the many symptoms it brings in your daily life.

Long term risks of PCOS:

Endometrial cancer- In American women, this is the most common reproductive cancer. Women with PCOS are at an increased risk for endometrial cancer because PCOS makes menstrual cycles occur very seldom for some women. Your chances of developing endometrial cancer increases if you have the following factors: obesity, infertility, hypertension or diabetes. (4) The most common symptoms associated with endometrial cancer are abnormal bleeding or vaginal discharge.

Ovarian Cancer- This is also known as the silent killer because it is rare to see any symptoms early on. Usually once they appear it has progressed to an untreatable stage. Ovarian cancer is the second most common gynecologic cancer and is most often seen in women who have had difficulty conceiving children. The risk of ovarian cancer is thought to be high for women with PCOS especially because of the ovulation induction medications. Symptoms associated with it are pain during intercourse, pain in the abdomen, swelling in the abdomen, abnormal vaginal bleeding, pelvic discomfort and gas, bloating or indigestion.

Heart disease- Women with PCOS have a high risk of developing heart disease mainly due to increased insulin levels. As discussed in other chapters, high insulin levels can increase many risks. In this case it can lead to high cholesterol and blood pressure. On top of that, being obese having a bad diet and exercise habits as well as smoking can lead to heart disease. Some warning symptoms to look for in heart disease are angina, fainting, edema, fatigue, palpitations and shortness of breath.

Miscarriage- PCOS women have a much higher chance for miscarriage than someone without PCOS. This is thought to be in part because PCOS causes longer menstrual cycles. With that comes a later ovulation date. The end result is the egg that is developing will be surrounded by a mass amount of hormones.

Diabetes- Type 2 diabetes is also known as adult onset diabetes. It is almost 20 times more common than type 1 diabetes (Juvenile).

Whether you have been recently diagnosed with PCOS or have had it for years, there is always more information out there to learn. It is incredibly easy to become confused, scared or even completely overwhelmed with it all. Hearing you've been diagnosed with anything you're unfamiliar with can send a jolt of fear down your spine. Fret not my fellow cyster. I'm here to help you make sense of Polycystic Ovarian Syndrome. This book is full of need to know facts about PCOS from one cyster to another.

Let's start at the beginning.

The prefix "Poly" means many. In layman terms Polycystic Ovarian Syndrome translates to: Many cysts on the ovaries

This is what a "normal" ovary looks like:

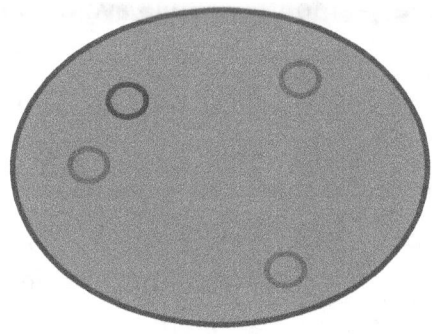

This is what a "polycystic" ovary looks like:

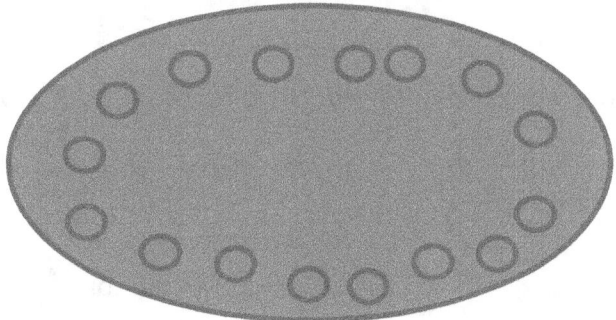

Have you ever heard the phrase "I'm so classy that even my ovaries wear pearls"? Well, now you see why. Polycystic ovaries basically look like a string of pearls has been wrapped around it.

In the case of PCOS, the term cyst is referring to a sac filled with fluid. Our "cysts" are actually follicles that began the process of maturation; however they didn't get released because no ovulation occurred. They then were left in the ovaries to form small and benign cysts.

The exact cause of PCOS is still unclear. There are some thoughts that it is hereditary. If your mother or sister has PCOS, your chance of developing it is increased.

Another thought is that PCOS develops when ovaries are exposed to levels of insulin that are too high, which is insulin resistance.

Whatever the cause may be, there is still not one clear test available to tell you 100% yes or no in regards to having PCOS. There are tests to verify symptoms and rule out other possibilities which will lead to a diagnosis of Polycystic Ovarian Syndrome.

After you have been diagnosed with PCOS, you'll want to sit down with your doctor and discuss a game plan to get it under control. Things that should be addressed to maintain your health are:

- Getting your period under control and regulated. (You want to have a menstrual cycle at least once every 3 months to help avoid endometrial cancer)
- Treating your infertility if you're wanting to try for children (You may need ovulation induction medication. PCOS can make it extremely difficult for women to become pregnant but by no means should the lack of ovulation be considered a substitute for birth control. Women with PCOS can spontaneously ovulate from time to time causing unwanted pregnancies.)
- Controlling insulin resistance (You may need medication or to create a diet and exercise plan)
- Eliminating long term risks such as diabetes, cancer, etc

There are a few different sets of criteria used to define PCOS. (5)

1.) Criteria from 1990 National Institutes of Health

- Hyperandrogenism
- Oligo-ovulation
- Exclusion of related disorders

2.) Criteria from 2003 Rotterdam

- Oligo- ovulation
- Hyperandrogenism
- Polycystic ovaries

3.) Criteria from 2006 Androgen Excess & PCOS Society

- Hyperandrogenism
- Anovulation, oligo- ovulation &/or Polycystic ovaries
- Exclusion of other androgen excess related disorders

Doctors typically look for 2 of the 3 characteristics when giving a diagnosis of Polycystic Ovarian Syndrome. The problem is that PCOS presents in every woman differently. This makes it difficult for some physicians to accurately diagnosis it. You'll see that not every set of criteria looks for polycystic ovaries. That is because the cysts are often "dissolved" by your body naturally. This means that they can be there one week and gone the next. There are also things out there that enable the cysts to disintegrate. Birth control pills are known to do this because most offer a dose of hormones that is pretty consistent. Certain herbs and alternative treatments have a similar effect. The cysts will come back though because our ovaries work "over time" so to speak, to over produce follicles.

FUN FACT

In 1809, Dr. Ephraim McDowell successfully removed a tumor from an ovary! Jane Crawford thought she was pregnant and carrying twins. After Dr. McDowell examined her, he became aware of the tumor. (5)

CHAPTER 2- PCOS SYMPTOM BREAKDOWN

Symptoms of PCOS

Most common PCOS symptoms are as follows:

- Acne
- Obesity (weight gain)
- Trouble losing weight
- Hirsutism
- Male Pattern Baldness
- Infertility
- Irregular Menstruation/No Menstruation/Heavy Menstruation
- Cysts on ovaries
- Insulin resistance

Other associated symptoms are as follows:

- Depression
- Deep voice
- Anxiety
- Sleep Apnea
- Dark patches on skin
- Skin tags
- High blood pressure
- High cholesterol
- Oily/dry skin
- Pelvic pain
- Dandruff

ACNE

Our skin is considered to be a direct reflection of the current health status of the inside of our body. Unfortunately for some, that is why certain groups of us suffer from severe acne while others have little to none. Seems fair, right?

Naturopaths believe that poor elimination of body wastes and toxins cause them to build up in our systems and then exit through our skin. The liver is the organ that is primarily responsible for detoxification. If it is bombarded with the wrong food or a hormonal imbalance, the end result will be acne. This happens because your liver won't be able to break things down and clear out the excess hormones from your body.

As teenagers most of us have been plagued with acne without much thought of possibly suffering from it as an adult. Below you will find multiple ways to possibly reduce the outbreak.

Acne is fairly easy to spot and comes in various forms: blackheads, whiteheads, red spots and even fluid filled lumps. In severe cases, scarring may occur.

Elevated androgen levels are the leading culprits behind acne, however there are other additional factors that can contribute to the development of acne. Stress, certain medications including oral contraceptives, hormonal imbalance, poor diet, genetics, allergies, and over washing your face can all lead to acne. Basically what happens, especially with women who have PCOS is androgen levels rise which causes dihydrotesterone (DHT) production to increase. DHT tells your body to make more oil which in turn can clog your pores enabling bacteria to get stuck in there thus creating pimples.

Medication:

o Trimethoprim	Tetracycline	Doxycycline	Minocycline
o Clindamycin	Azelaic Acid	Benzoyl Peroxide	
o Topical Retinoids			

Herbal Supplements:

o Saw Palmetto	Vitex	Red Clover	Alfalfa
o Yellow Dock Root	Calendula	Burdock Root	Hops
o Oregon Grape Root	Cayenne	Tea Tree Oil	Lady's Mantle
o Passionflower	Oregano Oil	Chamomile	Dandelion
o Lavender	Milk Thistle	Selenium	Vitamin B6
o Basil	Evening Primrose Oil		

Homeopathy:

- Sulphur   Silicea   Kalium Bromatum
- Calcarea Sulphurica   Hepar Suphuris Calcareum   Pulsatilla

Suggestions:

- Drink at least 8 glasses of water daily to keep system flushed
- Eat a high fiber diet. Fiber helps to cleanse the colon and remove toxins
- Switch to natural or water based cosmetics and creams
- Eat a high Zinc diet. Zinc is an antibacterial agent
- Keep area as oil free as possible
- Avoid alcohol, caffeine, chocolate, fried food, hot and spicy food
- Eliminate processed food
- Avoid stress
- Exercise
- Get sufficient sleep which is about 7-9 hours each night
- Don't pick at the pimples
- Do not scrub your face
- Wash your face twice daily with warm water and mild cleanser
- Take birth control which helps to balance hormones in turn reducing acne

Taking a nice warm steam bath with essential oils is such an excellent way to open up your pores. Not only are they great for oily or dry skin but they are so easy to do! Simply add a few drops of the essential oil of your liking to a bowl of freshly boiled water. Lower your face to the steam, cover your head and the bowl with a towel for 10-20 minutes.

- Oily skin- Cedarwood or lemongrass oil
- Dry skin- Rosewood, Rosemary or lavender

Another beneficial treatment is a face wash that you can do in the morning or evening. Get a shallow dish of water; add 20-30 drops of an herbal myrrh tincture and mix. Dab a cotton swab in it and clean your face using soft brush strokes.

OILY SKIN: This happens because sebaceous glands produce more oil than is required to keep skin lubricated. If your skin is oily, here are some essential oils that can help.

Juniper, Cedarwood, Ylang Ylang, Chamomile, Rosemary, Sandalwood, *Burdock Root, *Oat Straw, *Thyme, **Aloe Vera, ***Witch Hazel

*Help to nourish the skin, ** Has healing properties, *** Helps skin to absorb oil

DRY SKIN:

Cedarwood, Geranium, Sandalwood, Chamomile, Rosewood, Yarrow, Myrrh, Tea Tree, Rose, Jasmine, Neroli, Lavender, Aloe Vera, Calendula, *Comfrey

*Soothes irritated skin

Additional tips for dry skin:

- Eat a well-balanced diet.

- Moisturize after cleansing.

- Avoid extremely hot water. Stick to lukewarm water as hot water removes needed moisture from the skin.

- Drink about two quarts of water daily to keep skin hydrated.

- Avoid fried foods. Eat plenty of yellow and orange vegetables.

- Don't use harsh soaps.

HIRSUTISM

Hirsutism is abnormal or excessive facial or body hair growth on women. This is due to increased levels of androgens, which are the male hormones. Hirsutism usually appears as hair that is dark and course, growing on the upper legs, breasts, upper lip, upper arms, chest, face, back and lower abdomen. It is the most common indicator of hyperandrogenism and it affects approximately 8% of women in the USA, that's over 4 million women. (1)

In our day and age, society demands certain looks from us to fit their "norm". I know this, and you know this. It's no surprise how many women list hirsutism as their number two, if not, number one most hated symptom of PCOS, me included.

Let's face it; we have all had days where keeping up with our hair seems almost impossible. We wake up to stubble the next morning, I think most of us can relate. I've often compared my hair to my husbands and wondered how often he does the same.

Rest assured ladies, we do have options!

- Shaving. This is probably the most inexpensive choice. It does require the most time and upkeep.
- Waxing. One word → Ouch! I'll admit, I am not brave enough for this one. It can cause ingrown hairs, skin irritation, and redness. On the plus side it is fairly inexpensive and you do it in the privacy of your own home or go to a salon. It usually lasts for a week or two between waxing.
- Plucking. This is incredibly time consuming, painful and temporary. If you own tweezers, it's free and you can't beat that!
- Electrolysis. A permanent hair removal method that comes with plenty of drawbacks. It takes a lot of time to do a small area. It can also be very pain. Some say it is comparable to a bunch of shots or bee stings. The price tag is rather high and it may take multiple sessions and touch ups to get and or maintain the results you want. There is a possibility for burns, scarring and skin irritation.
- Bleaching. This is not a method for actual hair removal but rather hair lightening. It is not too expensive and you can do it at home. It does have the potential to cause skin irritation though.
- Laser Removal. The results are usually permanent. It is very expensive but can handle larger areas as opposed to electrolysis which only does a small section. It has been reported as being painful as well. Laser hair removal can cause irritation, scarring, burning and even loss of pigmentation at the treated sites.

If those options aren't what you are looking for, there are a few medication options to look into.

Medications:

- o   Topical Eflornithine   Birth Control   Spironolactone   Finasteride
- o   Flutamide

Herbal Supplements:

- o   Saw Palmetto   Vitex   Red Clover

SKIN TAGS

(Medical name: Acrochordon)

Much like the name implies, a skin tag is a small harmless piece of skin that hangs loosely, most commonly around the neck and armpit. Some might say they slightly resemble a balloon. Skin tags range in color from flesh tone to a dark brown. Skin tags are typically found in creases and thought to be the result of skin rubbing up against skin. They tend to grow on the eyelids, neck, armpits, folds of the groin, and under the breasts. They vary from person to person in size, location, amount and color. There is a strong relationship between obesity and skin tags.

There are many misconceptions about them, such as they are contagious, tumors or even that they grow back in increased numbers after removal.

Having them removed doesn't cause more to grow. They can be removed in many ways. Freezing them, cutting them, tying them off, and some even fall off on their own.

Aside from being uncomfortable, they don't pose other health risks.

ACANTHOSIS NIGRICANS

Most commonly known as the dark, velvety skin patches we notice around our armpits, neck and groin.

This is yet another embarrassing symptom of PCOS. Who wants dark patches on their body? Rhetorical question, the answer is obviously nobody.

This condition is not harmful nor does it pose any significant health risks. It is associated with insulin resistance.

Some things that might help are:

- Dermabrasion
- Laser Therapy
- Isotretinoin
- Creams containing Salicylic Acid or Alpha Hydroxy Acids

However the best way to get rid of it is to lower your insulin resistance with diet and exercise.

ALOPECIA

Alopecia is a partial or complete loss of hair usually caused by too much testosterone. Under "normal" conditions people lose about 50 to 100 hairs a day, however some medications do cause baldness as a side effect. For instance, Isotretinoin is a drug used to treat acne and known to cause baldness. Aside from medications, there are many other additional factors that can contribute to alopecia. Some of the causes are heredity, hormonal imbalance, pregnancy, menopause, stress, chemotherapy, crash diet, and nutritional deficiencies.

As cysters, we get double whammied in the hair department. It won't stay where it is supposed to and won't stay off where it is not supposed to be. Lucky for us, there are thousands of high quality fashionable wigs to be bought. Who doesn't like playing dress up?

If you prefer to stick with your own lovely locks, rest assured that there are medications available to help.

Medications:

- Minoxidil   Finasteride

Aromatherapy:

- Yarrow   Lemon Balm   Ylang Ylang   Rosemary
- Cedarwood   Clary Sage   Lavender

Suggestions:

- Avoid refined sugar, flour, saturated fat, and processed food as they impair circulation and deplete needed nutrients
- Exercise increases circulation
- Get 7-9 hours of sleep nightly
- Pat wet hair and gently squeeze remaining water out

CAM Treatments:

- Acupuncture   Massage   Relaxation   Yoga

Vitamins/Supplements:

- Vitamin E   Vitamin C   Iron   Gingko Biloba
- Biotin   Zinc   Saw Palmetto   Vitamin B Complex
- Tea Tree Oil

If your hair is oily add a couple drops per ounce of one of the following scents to your shampoo:

- Cedarwood   Cypress   Clary Sage   Bergamont

- Pine   Lemon   Juniper   Rosemary

- Tea Tree Oil   Geranium

If your hair is dry:

- Chamomile   Lavender   Rosemary

If you have dandruff:

Cedarwood	Atlas	Pine	Rosemary	Zinc
Sandalwood	Juniper	Thyme	Geranium	Lavender
Goldenseal	Dandelion	Tea Tree Oil	Red Clover	Selenium

Dandruff is the white flakes that are produced when dead skin on the head is shed. It is the old skin cells that are being shed. This can be caused by multiple conditions such as an illness, hormonal imbalance or nutritional deficiencies to name a few. Be sure to not scratch or pick at your scalp if you have dandruff.

SLEEP APNEA

Apnea means not breathing

PCOS increases the risk of having sleep apnea. Do you often wake up the next morning feeling abnormally tired, like you barely slept? It's possible you have sleep apnea and are completely unaware. It is usually spotted when you're snoring, stop and then gasp for air. Take a look at the following symptoms of sleep apnea.

- Loud snoring
- Depression
- Not breathing while sleeping
- Restless sleep
- Abnormal tiredness the next day
- Waking up tired
- Lethargy
- Poor concentration
- Awakening with dry mouth
- Morning headaches

If any of those sound familiar to you, talk to your doctor about the possibility of having sleep apnea. You can have a sleep study done to confirm the diagnosis. A sleep study is where you spend the night in a facility hooked up to painless monitors to see how you sleep and what happens. If you do in fact have sleep apnea, you will get a machine that can sit on your night stand. It hooks up to a small mask you wear over your mouth and nose during sleep to help you breath. This is called a CPAP machine which stands for continuous positive airway pressure. Sleep apnea should not be left untreated as it can lead to high blood pressure, heart arrhythmia and stroke.

Suggestions:

- You should avoid alcohol and sleeping pills
- Try sleeping on one side
- Stop smoking
- Lose weight
- Raise the head of the bed 4-6 inches
- Try acupuncture
- The flower essences Vervain has a calming effect

HIGH CHOLESTEROL

Cholesterol is viewed as LDL and HDL. HDL is referred as "good" cholesterol, while LDL is the "bad" cholesterol. HDL helps to clean up unneeded cholesterol that's in our blood vessel walls. It then takes it to the liver to be removed. LDL is referred to as bad because it enables the cholesterol to build up in our arteries which in turn can lead to heart disease.

Cholesterol is a fatty substance made in our liver. It does many good things when it is controlled. For instance, cholesterol is needed for our brains and nerves to function properly.

PCOS causes low HDL levels and high LDL levels, when we need it the other way around. There are many additional factors that could cause it to go up, such as: inactivity, stress, diabetes/insulin resistance, poor diet and hereditary. According to the National Heart, Lung and Blood Institute guidelines for cholesterol levels are as follows:

LDL LEVELS

Less than 100mg/dL	Optimal
100-129	Near/Less than optimal
130-159	Borderline high
160-189	High
Greater than or equal to 190	Very high

TOTAL CHOLESTEROL

Less than 200mg/dL	Desirable
200-239	Borderline high
Greater than or equal to 240	High

HDL LEVELS

Less than 40mg/dL	Low; major risk factor for heart disease
60mg/dL and above	Considered protective against heart disease

Symptoms of high cholesterol are: Dizziness, circulatory problems and mental confusion

Medications to help lower LDL levels:

- Statins (Like Lipitor)   Fibrates (Like Tricor)

Vitamins / Supplements:

- Magnesium   Vitamin E   Vitamin C   Garlic
- Artichoke Leaf   Shiitake Mushroom   Fenugreek Seed

Triglycerides are another kind of fat in our body, they're made from carbohydrates.

Suggestions to lower Triglycerides:

- Lose weight
- Avoid stress
- Reduce dietary fat and carbohydrate intake
- Reduce or avoid alcohol and caffeine intake
- Exercise
- Take Fish oil pills
- High fiber diet (Fruits, vegetables, whole grains)

Medications:

- Cholestryramine   Colestipol   Ezetimibe   Niacin
- Gemfibrozil   Neomycin   Raloxifene

Herbs:

- Cayenne   Goldenseal   Hawthorn   Cinnamon

HIGH BLOOD PRESSURE

High blood pressure is also known as the silent killer due to the fact the symptoms are easy to miss until complications arise. Some of those symptoms are nosebleeds, dizziness, ringing in the ears, blurred vision, headaches, sweating, flushed cheeks and shortness of breath. It is very easy for any of those to be blamed on other conditions. There are many other outside factors that could cause high blood pressure. It is very important to keep an eye on your blood pressure if you are obese, smoke, consume an excessive amount of alcohol, don't exercise, have diabetes or high cholesterol, anxiety or depression. If left untreated, high blood pressure can lead to heart disease, heart attack and strokes.

Your blood pressure is written as two numbers; a top number and bottom number. The top number is called systolic pressure, this is the pressure exerted by the blood when the heart beats. The systolic number typically ranges 90 - 120. The bottom number is called diastolic pressure and this number represents the heart resting between beats. This number should range 60-80.

Losing weight, dieting and exercise are all positive changes to help keep your blood pressure low. Other excellent suggestions are:

o   Lower salt intake. Avoid "Na" on food labels
o   Avoid the herb licorice as it can elevate blood pressure
o   Eat a high fiber diet with plenty of fruits and vegetables
o   Get regular aerobic exercise
o   Lower body weight by at least 10 pounds
o   Limit alcohol to one drink per day
o   Avoid caffeine
o   Get 7-9 hours of sleep nightly
o   Manage stress appropriately

If these changes don't help, you may need to start medication.

FUN FACT

Dark chocolate can help lower your blood pressure because it contains cocoa polyphenols.

Medications:

Beta Blockers:

- Acebutolol (Sectral)   Atenolol (Tenormin)

- Betaxolol (Kerlone)   Bisoprolol Fumarate (Zebeta)

- Carteolol Hydrochloride (Cartrol)   Metoprolol Tartrate (Lopressor)

- Metoprolol Succinate (Toprol-XL)   Nadolol (Corgard)

- Penbutolol Sulfate (Levatol)   Propranolol Hydrochloride (Inderal)

- Timolol Maleate (Blocadren)

ACE Inhibitors:

- Benazepril Hydrochloride (Lotensin)   Captopril (Capoten)

- Enalapril Maleate (Vasotec)   Fosinopril Sodium (Monopril)

- Lisinopril (Prinivel, Zestril)   Ramipril (Altace)

Herbs:

o Shepherds Purse	Alfalfa Leaf	Garlic	Cayenne
o Passion Flower*	Hawthorn**	California Poppy Root	Valerian*
o Dandelion***	Chamomile	Fennel	Parsley
o Rosemary	Hops*	Mistletoe	

*Relaxes nerves

**Dilates artery walls to decrease blood pressure

***Diuretic

CAM Treatments:

o Meditation	Yoga	Stretching	Walking
o Acupuncture	Aquatic Therapy	Tai Chi	Qigong

Essential Oils: Lavender, Marjoram, Ylang Ylang

Vitamins / Supplements:

- Calcium   Magnesium   Potassium   Vitamin E   CoQ-10
- Omega-3 Fatty Acid

Best foods for people with high blood pressure to eat are celery, garlic, onions, nuts, seeds, Coldwater fish, green leafy vegetables, whole grains, legumes, foods rich in vitamin c and flavonoids like cherries and grapes.

INSOMNIA

"Sleep is the golden chain that ties health and our bodies together" -Thomas Dekker 1572-1632

What many people might not know is there are two types of insomnia. Those two types are primary which means your insomnia isn't linked to other issues. Secondary insomnia is the second type and is the opposite of primary insomnia. It occurs as the result of another health issue like depression or pain.

A circadian biological clock located inside of the brain is what regulates sleep. A whole slew of problems can arise from lack of sleep. It affects the cardiovascular and immune system as well as can cause obesity and gastrointestinal problems. There are many reasons sleep cycles can be interrupted. The top factors are caffeine, nicotine, alcohol and sugar. Additional factors are stress, lack of exercise, anxiety, restless leg syndrome (R.L.S), asthma, sleep apnea, hormonal imbalance, pain, medicine, and blood sugar instability.

Ideally 8 hours of sleep is recommended each night. Only about 35% of Americans meet that quota. As humans, we go nonstop without much thought about sleep or lack thereof.

Symptoms of insomnia: Difficulty falling asleep, waking in the middle of the night or too early in the morning, feeling tired after a full night's sleep, daytime irritability or fatigue.

Tips to sleep better:

- Stay active but avoid exercise 5-6hours before bedtime. Exercise causes your body temperature to rise and then fall many hours later.

- Follow a bedtime routine as well as getting up and going to bed at the same time if possible
- Limit caffeine and alcohol close to bedtime. Caffeine takes around 3-5 hours to leave your body
- Allow sufficient time to unwind
- No large meals within two hours of bedtime
- Hide alarm clock to avoid minute counting
- Create a comfortable sleep space
- Don't force sleep
- Avoid naps or limit to 30 minutes or less
- Epsom salt soaks help relax muscles
- Help restore the clock in your body by darkening your home about 1 hour before bed. This will help melatonin production.
- Avoid bacon, cheese, ham, potatoes, sugar, spinach and tomatoes close to bedtime. (They contain tyramine which releases norepinephrine which is a brain stimulant)

Keeping a sleep diary is an excellent way to track your sleep and why you may be having problems with insomnia. Write down things like:

- Any medications you are taking at the time

- What time you went to sleep and what time you woke up

- How many times you woke during the night and for how long

- What you ate or drank last and at what time

- What emotions or stress you had throughout the day

CAM Treatments:

- Relaxation   Acupuncture   Aromatherapy   Massage
- Exercise   Yoga   Chiropractor

Essential Oils:

- Bergamont   Cypress   Geranium   Jasmine   Lavender
- Melissa   Lemonbalm   Neroli   Chamomile   Rose
- Sandalwood   Vetiver   Yarrow   Ylang Ylang

Homeopathy:

- Avena Stiva,   Nux Vomica,   Coffea,   Kalium Phosphoricum
- Calcarea Carbonica,   Kalium Bromatum,   Nux Moschata

Herbs to try:

- Feverfew   California Poppy   Hops   Skullcap
- Chamomile   Kava   Lavender   Valerian
- Catnip   Passionflower   Lemon Balm   Basil
- Bergamont   Dandelion   Marjoram
- Evening Primrose Oil   St. John's Wort

Vitamins/Minerals to try:

- B3 (Niacin)   B6 (Pyridoxine)   Calcium   Magnesium

*B3 and B6 trigger the production of tryptophan and serotonin which are natural chemicals that help people sleep. Try eating bananas, dates, figs, turkey, whole grain and milk close to bed as they're all high in tryptophan.

Medications:

- Barbiturates   Melatonin   Ramelteon
- Benzodiazepines   Triazolam   Zolpidem
- Eszopiclone   Zolpiclone   Meprobamate
- Trazodone   Zaleplon

DEPRESSION

There is no doubt in any cysters mind about how much we endure every day. It is possible to become depressed along the way. PCOS women are at a greater risk of becoming depressed. It is nothing to be ashamed about. There are many things that could cause depression such as stress, chemical imbalance, traumatic event, poor diet, nutritional deficiencies, medications, chronic illness, alcohol, drugs, sleep disturbance, genetics, isolation, etc. This is a real problem, not something made up in your head. It does not mean you are weak my fellow cyster.

I'm sure a good portion of us have experienced some of the symptoms below.

- Feeling sad, down, hopeless or worthless
- Crying for no reason
- Loss of interest in daily activities &/or sex
- Sleeping problems or restlessness
- Difficulty focusing, concentrating or making decisions.
- Irritability
- Unusual fatigue or weakness
- Unexplained weight gain
- Unintentional weight loss
- Unexplained physical symptoms- back pain, headaches, or no appetite.

There is help available to you. Always remember, you are NOT alone in this battle.

Herbs:

- Lemon Balm   Ginger   Ginkgo Biloba   Licorice Root   Kava
- Oat Straw   Peppermint   St John's Wart   Rose
- Rosemary   Skullcap   Wormwood   Mugwort
- Raspberry   Feverfew   Jasmine   Lavender

Vitamins/ Supplements:

- Folate   St. John's Wart   DHEA   Selenium
- Ginseng   Omega-3 Fatty Acid   Reishi

Medications

Tricyclic Anti-Depressants:

- Amitriptyline (Elavil)   Desipramine (Norpramin)

- Nortriptyline (Pamelor, Aventyl)
- Trimipramine (Surmontil)

Tetracyclics:

- Maprotiline (Cudiomil)   Mirtazapine (Remeron)

MAOI's:

- Isocarboxazid (Marplan)   Phenelzine (Nardil)
- Tranylaypromine (Parnate)

Stimulants:

- Methylphenidate (Ritalin, Concerta)   Dextramphetamine (Dexedrine, Dextrostat)
- Modafinil (Provigil)   Lithium (Eskalith, Lithobid)

CAM Treatments:

- Guided imagery   Acupuncture   Reiki   Massage
- Relaxation   Hypnotherapy   Meditation   Aromatherapy
- Flower Essences   Supplements

Suggestions:

- Stay active
- Avoid alcohol as it blocks the absorption of Vitamin B
- Eat 5-6 smaller meals daily
- Avoid caffeine and refined sugar

Essential Oils:

- Cedarwood   Bergamont   Cypress   Frankincense   Geranium
- Grapefruit   Jasmine   Juniper   Lavender   Lemongrass
- Lemonbalm   Myrrh   Neroli   Chamomile   Rose
- Rosemary   Yarrow   Vetiver   Melissa   Ylang Ylang
- Sandalwood   Sweet Marjoram

Homeopathy:

- Natrum Muriaticum Sepia Lachesis Pulsatilla
- Aurum Metallicum

ANXIETY

The word anxiety comes from the Latin word "angere" which means to choke or strangle. Often anxiety accompanies depression. It can be a painful event psychologically when it happens. Apprehension strikes and you have trouble concentrating. A feeling of dread goes through your body, you become irritable and agitated. Your heart rate increases, it's hard to breathe, your palms become sweaty, but why?

There are a number of probable factors: fears, conflicts or extreme phobias. Sometimes anxiety can be good because it pushes us to better ourselves, like speaking in front of crowds.

Symptoms:

- Elevated blood pressure, increased muscle tension, rapid or difficulty breathing, rapid heart rate, disturbed sleep patterns, nausea, upset stomach, dizziness, headache, chest pain, heart palpitations, sweaty palms, restlessness, trembling, trouble concentrating,

Having PCOS, our anxiety is caused from a hormonal imbalance. However there are many other outside factors that could cause anxiety issues. Some additional causes are stress, the environment, poor nutrition, thyroid issues, low blood sugar, depression, adrenal disorder, allergies, disturbed sleep, medications, alcohol, drugs, caffeine, nicotine and even simply genetics.

There are things that can help.

- Eat diet of apricots, asparagus, avocados, bananas, broccoli, brown rice, figs, fish, garlic, green leafy vegetables, raw nuts, whole grain and yogurt. Stress can deplete levels of calcium, magnesium, phosphorus and potassium which these foods can replenish
- Eat complex carbs such as brown rice and oats. They contain serotonin which has a calming effect on the brain
- Avoid alcohol and caffeine
- Avoid refined sugars. Chromium deficiencies have the ability of producing symptoms that resemble anxiety such as shaking, nervousness, etc.
- Learn relaxation techniques
- Regular Exercise
- Have a support system to call

CAM Treatments:

- Deep breathing   Meditation   Hypnosis   Relaxation
- Visualization   Stretching   Walking   Acupuncture

- Aromatherapy   Flower Essences

Supplements:

- Calcium   Fish Oil   Selenium   Magnesium
- Vitamin B

Herbs:

- California poppy root   St John's Wort   Passionflower   Valerian
- Chamomile   Crampbark   Hops   Kava
- Motherwort   Catnip   Lemonbalm   Basil
- Evening Primrose Oil   Lavender   Marjoram   Skullcap
- Valerian   Wormwood   Jasmine

Homeopathy:

- Ignatia   Aconite   Argentum Nitricum   Calcarea
- Carbonica   Arsenicum Album

An activity called systematic desensitization helps with anxiety by confronting the underlying fears and phobias. For example; if you're feeling anxious about an upcoming ivf treatment, you would envision yourself going and getting through it perfectly fine.

The biggest thing to remember when you're experiencing an anxiety attack is focus on calm breathing. When you constantly do not have enough oxygen it can make many issues that much worse. Symptoms like stress, asthma, phobias, headaches, high blood pressure and anxiety are increased. Rapid shallow breathing tightens blood vessels.

Essential oils such as Vanilla, Geranium and Bergamont can help. Simply put 2 or 3 drops of the oil of your choice on a cotton ball and gently smell.

TREATMENT FOR DEPRESSION & ANXIETY

Herbs:

- Kava   St. John's Wort   Valerian   Ginkgo Biloba
- Passionflower   Chamomile   Ginger

Supplements:

- Omega-3 Fatty Acid
- Vitamin C
- Calcium

Vitamin B Complex
Vitamin D
Manganese

Folate
Magnesium
Iron

SSRI's & SNRI's:

SSRI's (Selective Serotonin Reuptake Inhibitors) are the most commonly prescribed type of medication as they tend to work more effectively without causing addictions. The biggest drawback to this type of medication is that they can take 2 to 4 weeks before you see any improvement. Unfortunately many people stop taking their medications during this time thinking that it really isn't helping. SNRI'S are Serotonin and norepinephrine reuptake inhibitors. They are not habit forming. Common side effects are:

- Drowsiness
- Sleep problems
- Weight loss or gain

Dizziness
Vivid & strange dreams
Changes in appetite

Headache
Sexual problems

SNRI's:

- Duloxetine (Cymbalta)

venlafaxine (Effexor)

SSRI's:

- Citalopram (Celexa)
- Fluvoxamine (Luvox)

Escitalopram (Lexapro)
Paroxetine (Paxil)

Fluoxetine (Prozac)
Sertraline (Zoloft)

Benzodiazepines:

- Alprazolam (Xanax and Xanax XR)
- Diazepam (Valium)
- Halazepam (Paxipam)

Clonazepam (Klonopin)
Lorazepam (Ativan)

Eating foods that are rich in tryptophan can increase production of serotonin. Example: Dairy, eggs, soy beans.

Vitamins:

- o   Vitamin B Complex   Calcium   Magnesium   Inositol

Herbs:

- o   California Poppy Root   Valerian   Kava   Lavender

OBESITY

Your level of obesity will be measured with what is called a BMI chart. This stands for Body Mass Index. BMI charts enable doctors to determine your body fat. What they do is take your weight and height and calculate to get a number, your BMI.

Underweight: Less than 18.5

Normal weight: 18.5 to 24.9

Overweight: 25.0 to 29.9

Obese: 30.0 or greater

It's no secret that PCOS makes it much harder to lose weight than women without PCOS. As a matter of fact, approximately 50% of women with PCOS are overweight. (2) However it is thought that losing just 5-7% of your current body weight could help to reduce many of the symptoms PCOS has to offer.

That is a small goal to start with, although for some it could be viewed as a very daunting task. There are some excellent resources listed in further chapters that can help get you going. After all, weight loss does so much good for our bodies including decreasing testosterone levels, insulin resistance, risk of cardiovascular disease and diabetes. It can also improve our menstrual cycle and bring more regularity to it and ovulation.

Losing weight before you conceive will not only help you to conceive but also reduce your risks of getting gestational diabetes and hypertension. Obese pregnant women also have a high risk of being induced, having longer labors, requiring c-sections or having complications following delivery.

Always remember to NOT starve yourself in an attempt to lose weight.

Auricular acupuncture is said to help regulate appetite.

Herbs with diuretic properties:

- Alfalfa Dandelion Hyssop Juniper Oat Straw Parsley Thyme Yarrow

INFERTILITY

There are so many factors that can contribute to infertility. A few of the most common conditions are:

- PCOS - #1 most common condition causing infertility in women

- Endometriosis

- Pelvic Inflammatory Disease (PID)

- Premature Ovarian Failure

Infertility can bring about a whole mess of feelings; denial (the tests are wrong), guilt (it's all my fault), isolation (no one understands what I'm going through), indifference (why can't I get pregnant easily like her), frustration (why won't it work), despair (I'll never have a baby), not to mention anger, depression, irritability, anxiety and a mourning for a child you may never have. Infertility is not fun, nor is it fair. No one deserves it. It doesn't discriminate. Infertility doesn't care what your educational level is, how old you are, what race you are, if you have conceived before, what your profession is or even your income level. In the eyes of infertility, we are all the same.

You didn't chose to have this struggle with infertility but you can chose how to react to it. By accepting you can't control everything, learning to let go and setting expectations that are reasonable and realistic, you can become empowered.

So many other factors can affect your fertility; stress, alcohol, tobacco, STD's, vitamin deficiencies, anxiety, caffeine, underweight, overweight or low thyroid function to name a few.

Infertility is defined as the inability to become pregnant after one year of sexual activity without contraception.

How many times have you been asked about your family situation; are you married, do you have kids? Both are such innocent questions for the average person. For women with PCOS who are infertile, it is filled with memories of charting, medications, appointments, even relationship problems and scheduled sex.

Medications:

- Bromocriptine   Clomiphene   Danazol   Progestins

Herbs:

- Vitex   Black Cohosh   Dong Quai   Motherwort

CAM Treatments:

- Acupuncture   Relaxation   Reflexology   Reiki

Homeopathy:

- Sepia   Aristolochia   Oophorinum   Folliculinum
- Kalium   Carbonicum

Suggestions:

- Eliminate caffeine and smoking
- Eat a balanced diet
- Add nutritional supplements
- Eat plenty of pineapple cores. The hard fibrous middle part contains an enzyme called bromelain which helps implantation by making the uterine lining thicker and stickier for the egg to latch on.
- Get plenty of Vitamin E. In 1922 Vitamin E was named "Fertility Factor X" because the laboratory rats used needed it to reproduce. A few years later it was renamed as "Tocopherol" from the Greek word Tocos which means "childbirth."

We don't usually give much thought to radiation from common household objects and how it interferes with our body.

o   Don't use the cell phone when the battery is low. Don't put the cell phone to your ear until the other party answers because the signal is the strongest while ringing.

o   Try using a desktop computer instead of a laptop. We typically put a laptop on our laps, right? Our lap is so close to our reproductive organs.

o   Don't sit too close to the television as it gives off radiation.

o   If it's possible, leave the kitchen while using appliances such as the microwave, oven, blender, etc. If it's in use, it is giving off radiation.

o   Try moving your bed away from the bedroom wall to avoid the energy coursing through the walls.

MENSTRUAL CYCLES

Herbs to help irregular menstruation:

o Angelica	Dill	Basil	Marigold	Feverfew	Gentian
o Hops	Mugwort	Raspberry	Rose	Skullcap	
o Fennel	Strawberry	Carrot	Beets(raw, juice, powder)		

Drugs to help with amenorrhea:

o   Bromocriptine   Progestins

PROFUSE BLEEDING

Causes:

o Fibroids	Uterine polyps	Endometriosis	Underactive thyroid
o IUD	Overweight		

Herbs:

o Lemon Juice	Lentil	Red Raspberry	Thyme
o Cayenne Pepper	Cinnamon Bark	Shepherds Purse	Lady's Mantle
o Yarrow	Seaweed		

Medications:

o   Antifibrinolytic Agents   Danazol   Estrogens   Progestins

Supplements:

- Iron   Folic Acid   Vitamin A   Vitamin C

There are many reasons why menstrual cycles may become irregular.

Symptoms:

- Stress   Prolactin Issues   Anorexia   Premature Menopause
- Thyroid Disease   Adrenal Gland Issues

Homeopathy:

- Calcarea Phosphoricum   Kali Carbonica   Natrum Muriaticum

CAM Treatment:

- Acupuncture   Exercise

Essential Oils:

- Clary Sage   Juniper   Lavender   Melissa   Lemon Balm
- Myrrh   Chamomile   Rose   Rosemary   Sweet Fennel
- Sweet Marjoram   Yarrow

MENSTRUAL CRAMPS

Causes:

- Stress   Genetics   Endometriosis   Fibroids
- Pelvic Inflammation Disease

Drugs:

- NSAIDS

Supplements:

- Magnesium   Pyridoxine (B6)   Vitamin E   Calcium   Iron

CAM Treatment:

- Massage   Chiropractor*   Relaxation   Guided Imagery
- Yoga   Acupressure   Acupuncture   Aromatherapy

*Chiropractors can offer spinal manipulation which is said to relieve menstrual cramps.

Herbs:

- Black Haw   Cinnamon   Cat nip   Chamomile   Valerian
- Kava   Garlic   Calendula   Marjoram   Crampbark
- Black Cohosh   Vitex   Willow   Evening Primrose Oil
- St John's Wort   Yellowdock   Rose   Peppermint

Suggestions:

- Hot water bottle/warm bath/heating pad

Homeopathy:

- Chamomilla   Megnesia Phosphoricum   Nux Vomica
- Viburnum Opulus   Cactus Gandiflorus   Kalium Carbonicum

Essential Oils:

- Clary Sage   Cypress   Juniper   Lavender   Sweet Fennel
- Sweet Marjoram   Vetiver

PMS

If you ask 20 women what PMS is like, you'll get 20 different answers.

Causes:

- High sugar diet   Caffeine   Genetics

Supplements:

- Magnesium   Calcium   Pyridoxine (B6)   Manganese

- Vitamin E   Zinc   Vitamin B

Herbs:

- Evening Primrose Oil   Dandelion Root*   Ladys Mantle**
- Angelica   Cramp Bark   Kava
- Passion Flower   Black Cohosh   False Unicorn Root
- Fennel   Black Haw   Rosemary
- Strawberry Leaf   Valerian   Wild Yam
- Yarrow   St John's Wort   Vitex
- Peppermint   Raspberry   Milk Thistle
- Feverfew   Skullcap   Dong Quai

*Regulates estrogen levels by helping liver to remove excess estrogen

**Ladys mantle (Alchemilla Vulgaris) helps controls heavy bleeding during menstruation.

FUN FACT

"alchemilla" means magic

Medications:

- NSAIDS   Danazol   SSRI's   Buspirone

Essential Oils:

- Frankincense   Geranium   Grapefruit   Lavender   Neroli   Rose
- Lemon Balm   Chamomile   Sandalwood   Vetiver   Bergamont
- Clary Sage   Jasmine   Juniper   Cypress   Rosemary
- Sweet Fennel

The symptoms of PMS usually begin one to two weeks before aunt flow arrives. While they vary, the most common symptoms are:

- Acne   Constipation/Diarrhea   Bloating   Emotional Changes
- Fatigue   Tension Anxiety   Aggression   Poor Concentration
- Weakness   Breast Tenderness   Cramps   Depression
- Irritability   Insomnia   Headache   Cravings Increased appetite

Suggestions:

- Eat plenty of fruits, vegetables, whole grain cereals, and high protein snacks between meals
- Diets high in fiber help to rid body of excess estrogen
- Try increasing water intake to 1 quart daily one week before period up to one week after
- No salt, junk food or fast foods at least one week before period
- Avoid caffeine
- Limit dairy
- Regular exercise

Homeopathy:

- Lachesis   Natrum Muriaticum   Nux Vomica   Pulsatilla Sepia

CAM Treatments:

- Acupuncture   Exercise   Guided Imagery   Massage
- Relaxation   Reflexology   Yoga

INSULIN RESISTANCE

To understand this, you must first understand insulin. It is produced by the pancreas. The pancreas is a gland close to your stomach. Not only does it secrete the protein hormones insulin and glucagon, it also releases enzymes to help digestion and absorption of dietary sugars. When you eat, your sugar levels rise and insulin is released to reduce the amount of glucose in your blood. When you are insulin resistant, you need to release higher levels of insulin. When you skip a lot of meals you increase the chance of developing insulin resistance. There are many other additional risk factors such as; family history of type 2 diabetes, hypertension, coronary vascular disease, getting older, lack of exercise and having PCOS.

Signs of insulin resistance are:

- High triglyceride levels
- High blood pressure
- Increased risk of cardiovascular disease
- Skin condition called acanthosis nigricans
- Increased ovarian production of androgens
- Infrequent ovulations
- Increased serum androgens
- Lowered liver production of SHBG
- Large waist circumference

In 2003 the criteria was established by the American Association of Clinical Endocrinologists (AACE) to diagnose insulin resistance syndrome. It is as follows: (3)

- BMI of 25 or higher
- Triglyceride level of 150mg/dL or higher
- Hdl level of 50mg/dL or less
- Blood pressure of 130/85 or more
- A 2 hour glucose level or 140mg/dL or more
- A fasting glucose level between 110 and 125 mg/dL

*A normal fasting blood glucose level should fall in the range of 65-99mg/dL

As I'm sure you can imagine, being insulin resistant can lead to a whole slew of problems. Did you know that higher insulin levels can negatively affect the quality of our eggs? It sure can. Not only that, higher insulin levels raise testosterone levels which can interfere with implantation. How scary is that? Here are a few more reasons to get your insulin levels under control, just in case that wasn't enough. If you conceive and are insulin resistant, you increase your chances of getting gestational diabetes, pre-eclampsia and pregnancy induced hypertension. You may have excessive weight gain. It's possible to deliver preterm and need a C-section because you're having a larger baby.

By now you should see that everything in our body is intertwined. Every hormone, nutrient, and system is all connected and the slightest upset in one area will cause chaos in another area.

For instance; not getting enough sleep stimulates cortisol to be released in higher amounts which makes your insulin levels go up.

High levels of cortisol encourage your body to store its weight around your midsection.

FUN FACT

<u>Drinking alcohol stimulates cortisol to be released thus gaining weight around the middle and earning the name "beer belly"</u>

High insulin levels also increase inflammation (acne). We need to always have a minimum level of glucose in our blood stream. This is essential for our brain and central nervous system (CNS) to function properly. When your glucose level drops too low, we experience hypoglycemia. Symptoms include dizziness, nausea, and trembling, incoherent and rambling speech.

Supplements to help lower glucose levels:

o Alpha lipoic acid	Vitamin B Complex	Biotin
o Chromium Picolinate	CLA	Coenzyme Q-10
o Magnesium	Manganese	Taurine
o Vitamin C	Vitamin D	Vitamin E
o Inositol	Calcium	Zinc

*taurine levels lower with stress

Herbs:

o Fenugreek	Gymnema	Sylvestre	Cinnamon
o Black Cohosh	Vitex		

CHAPTER 3- MEDICATIONS USED WITH PCOS

Polycystic Ovarian Syndrome is not the worst thing out there; however it is not the best either. It's pretty safe to assume once diagnosed, over the course of your life you will be prescribed some type of medication. Whatever it may be for, you have the right to know all about it. Whenever you get a new prescription be sure to ask:

- Generic and brand name of medication
- What is it for
- How many should you take and how often
- How should it make you feel
- What side effects to expect
- How to take it (with food, etc)
- How long will you be on it
- What happens if you miss a dose
- Food, drinks, other medications to avoid while on it
- Activity restrictions while on this
- What to do if symptoms don't change
- When to seek help
- How to store the medication and what to do with unused medications
- Expiration date
- Medication cost
- How many refills and when to refill
- If you're trying to get pregnant, will this medication cause any harm if you happen to conceive

Remember brand names can come with a large price tag. Do not be shy about asking for generics. They are much less expensive and work just as well.

Medications listed by disorder:

Anxiety:

- Xanax (Alprazolam)   Buspar (Buspirone)   Valium (Diazepam)

- Atarax, Vistaril (Hydroxyzine)   Ativan (lorazepam)   Serax (Oxazepam)

- Paxil (Paroxetine)   Desyrel (Trazodone)   Effexor (Venlafaxine)

Depression:

- Elavil, Endep (Amitriptyline)   Wellbutrin (Bupropion)   Celexa (Citalopram)
- Anafranil (Clomipramine)   Norpramin (Desipramine)   Pristiq (Desvenlafaxine)
- Sinequan (Doxepin)   Cymbalta (Duloxetine)   Lexapro (Escitalopram)
- Prozac (Fluoxetine)   Luvox (Fluvoxamine)   Fetzima (Levomilnacipram)
- Tofranil (Imipramine)   Ludiomil (Maprotiline)   Remeron (Mirtazapine)
- Aventyl, Pamelor (Nortriptyline)   Paxil (Paroxetine)   Nardil (Phenelzine)
- Emsam (Selegiline)   Zoloft (Sertraline)   Parnate (Tranylcypromine)
- Desyrel (Trazodone)   Effexor (Venlafaxine)   Brintellix (Vortioxetene)

High Cholesterol:

- Lipitor (Atorvastatin)   Questran (Cholestyramine)   Welchol (Colesevelam)
- Colestid (Colestipol)   Zetia (Ezetimibe)   Tricor (Fenofibrate)
- Lovaza (Fish Oil)   Lescol (Fluvastatin)   Lopid (Gemfibrozil)
- Niaspan (Niacin)   Crestor (Rosuvastatin)   Zocor (Simvastatin)

Hypertension:

- Norvasc (Amlodipine)   Tenormin (Atenolol)   Edarbi (Azilsartan)
- Lotensin (Benazepril)   Zebeta (Bisoprolol)   Capoten (Captopril)
- Catapres (Clonidine)   Vasotec (Enalapril)   Teveten (Eprosartan)
- Monopril (Fosinopril)   Lozol (Indapamide)   Avapro (Irbesartan)
- Zestril (Lisinopril)   Zaroxolyn (Metolazone)   Lopressor (Metoprolol)
- Loniten (Minoxidil)   Propranolol (Inderal)   Altace (Ramipril)
- Diovan (Valsartan)   Isoptin (Verapamil)

Insomnia:

- Benadryl (Diphenhydramine)   ProSom (Estazolam)   Lunesta (Eszopiclone)

- Dalmane (Flurazepam)   Rozerem (Ramelteon)   Sonata (Zaleplon)

- Ambien (Zolpidem)

Obesity:

- Didrex (Benzphetaine)   Wellbutrin (Bupropion)   Alli (Orlistat)

Generic name: Metformin   Brand name: Glucophage
Uses: Insulin resistance, Type 2 Diabetes. Metformin can help to restore regular menstrual cycles and fertility by controlling insulin resistance
Notes: Metformin has been known to deplete levels of Vitamin B12.
Side effects: Diarrhea, flatulence, nausea, upset stomach

Generic name: Clomiphene Citrate   Brand name: Clomid, Serophene
Uses: Ovulation induction, regulate cycles, increase egg production, correct luteal phase deficiency
Side effects: hot flashes, mood disturbances, headaches, nausea, breast tenderness, visual disturbances, and hyper stimulation syndrome (OHSS).
Notes: Originally discovered in 1956. This drug can cause hostile cervical mucus.

Generic name: Elfornithine   Brand name: Vaniga
Uses: Prescription skin cream to slow hair growth
Side effects: Acne, rash, stinging skin
Notes: Not a permanent solution as the hair will regrow once the cream is discontinued. It doesn't "remove" the hair, only slows growth and decreases length.

Generic name: Medroxyprogesterone   Brand name: Provera
Uses: Secondary amenorrhea, abnormal uterine bleeding from a hormonal imbalance
Side effects: Acne, hair loss, irritability, nervousness, insomnia, weight gain, anxiety, dizziness

Generic name: Letrozole   Brand name: Femara

Uses: Ovulation induction

Side effects: Irritability, nervousness, increased appetite, nausea, constipation, fatigue, hot flashes, abdominal pain

Generic name: Spironolactone   Brand name: Aldactone

Uses: Alopecia, Acne, Hirsutism, Edema

Side effects: Nausea, headache, diarrhea, abdominal cramps, fever, breast tenderness, vomiting

Notes: Diuretic that lowers androgen levels

Generic name: Clindamycin   Brand name: Cleocin

Uses: Bacterial infections, acne

Side effects: Dry skin, red and irritated skin

Notes: More commonly prescribed as a topical antibiotic in foam, gel or lotion form.

Generic name: Minoxidil (Topical)   Brand name: Rogaine

Uses: Alopecia

Side effects: Itching and dryness of scalp

Notes: Minoxidil is used topically on scalp. Hair loss will return once medication is stopped.

Generic name: Minoxidil (Systemic)   Brand name: Loniten

Uses: High blood pressure

Side effects: Breast tenderness, headache, edema

Generic name: Finasterida   Brand name: Propecia

Uses: Hirsutism

Side effects: Upset stomach, headache, dry skin

Notes:: Anti-androgenic medication that works by blocking testosterone from turning into androgens. Finasteride should not be used while pregnant as it can cause feminine characteristics in a male fetus. The herb St. John's Wort may reduce the concentration of Propecia.

Generic name: Minocycline   Brand name: Dynacin, Minocin
Uses: Acne
Side effects: Dizziness, diarrhea, nausea, fatigue, abdominal cramps
Notes: Antibiotic. The herbs Dong Quai and St. John's Wort may increase the risk of developing photo sensitivity while on Minocycline.

Generic name: Erythromycin   Brand name: Eryc, Ery-Tab
Uses: Skin infections, pelvic inflammatory infections, UTI, acne
Side effects: Diarrhea, vomiting, stomach pains, headache, fatigue
Notes: Be sure to wear sunscreen while using this medication as it makes skin more sensitive to sunlight.

Generic name: Doxycycline   Brand name: Adoxa, Oracea, Vibramycin
Uses: Acne, PID, respiratory infections
Side effects: Nausea, vomiting
Notes: This medication may decrease the effects of oral birth control

TRICYCLIC ANTI DEPRESSANTS
Generic name: Amitriptyline   Brand name: Elavil
Generic name: Clomipramine   Brand name: Anafranil
Generic name: Desipramine   Brand name: Norpramin
Generic name: Imipramine   Brand name: Tofranil
Generic name: Nortriptyline   Brand name: Pamelor
Uses: Depression, anxiety, OCD, ADHD, smoking cessation
Side effects: Drowsiness, constipation, fatigue, headache, nausea, dizziness, dry mouth

Azelaic Acid
Generic name: None available   Brand name: Azelex, Finevin, Finacea
Uses: Acne (Topical)
Side effects: Peeling, itching, redness, dryness of skin
Notes: May cause hypopigmentation in women with complexions that are darker. It may take a couple months to notice changes.

Benzoyl Peroxide
Uses: Acne
Side effects: Mild redness, skin irritation, chapping during first few weeks of use
Notes: Active ingredient in most soaps, lotions and cleaners. It is used topically to clear away bacteria from the skin.

Generic name: Bromocriptine Brand name: Cycloset
Uses: Ovulation induction, regulates menstrual cycle, breast pain, type 2 diabetes, PMS
Side effects: Dizziness, mild nausea, light headed, headache, constipation, diarrhea, tiredness, drowsiness, dry mouth, depression

Generic name: Buspirone Brand name: Buspar
Uses: Anxiety, PMS
Side effects: Nausea, Headache, Dizziness, Insomnia, Diarrhea, Dry Mouth

Generic name: Flutamide Brand name: Euflex
Uses: Hirsutism
Side effects: Hot flashes, diarrhea, nausea
Notes: Anti-Androgenic medication that blocks androgen receptors. The herb St. John's Wort may decrease the concentration of this medication.

Generic name: Danazol Brand name: Cyclomen, Danocrine
Uses: Pelvic pain, infertility, breast pain
Side effects: Weight gain, hot flashes, vaginal dryness, voice hoarseness
Notes: Anti-Androgenic medication that works by reducing the amount of hormones that are made by the ovaries.

Generic name: Clonazepam Brand name: Klonopin
Uses: Anxiety, panic disorders
Side effects: Dizziness, irritability, constipation

Generic name: Diazepam Brand name: Valium
Uses: Anxiety, panic disorders
Side effects: Fatigue, drowsiness, headache, nausea

Generic name: Lorazepam Brand name: Ativan
Uses: Anxiety, insomnia
Side effects: Drowsiness, nausea, headache

Generic name: Alprazolam Brand name: Xanax
Uses: Anxiety, panic disorders, depression
Side effects: Drowsiness, headache, nausea, diarrhea, light headedness
Notes: The herb St. John's Wort can decrease the effectiveness of this medication.
Generic name: Eszopiclone Brand name: Lunesta

Uses: Insomnia
Side effects: Dry mouth, diarrhea, headache

Generic name: Isotretinoin   Brand name: Absorica, Amnesteem, Claravis
Uses: Acne
Side effects: Nausea

MAOI's
Generic name: Phenelzine   Brand name: Nardil
Generic name: Tranylcypromine   Brand name: Parnate
Uses: Depression
Side effects: Weight gain

Generic name: Lithium   Brand name: Duralith, Lithobid
Uses: Depression, mood stabilizer
Side effects: Mild tremors, nausea, weight gain

Generic name: Mirtazapine   Brand name: Remeron, Remeron Soltab
Uses: Depression
Side effects: Drowsiness, dry mouth, weight gain, constipation

Generic name: Nefazodone   Brand name: Serzone
Uses: Depression
Side effects: Strange dreams, constipation, dry mouth

Generic name: Progesterone   Brand name: Prochieve, Prometrium
Uses: menstrual/uterine disorders, contraceptive, menopause, hormone imbalance, infertility from progesterone deficiency, amenorrhea
Side effects: Drowsiness, edema, weight gain, breast tenderness

Generic name: Scopolamine   Brand name: Hyoscine
Uses: Painful menstruation
Side effects: Dry mouth, headache

SSRI'S

Generic name: Lexapro	Brand name: Escitalopram
Generic name: Zoloft	Brand name: Sertraline
Generic name: Celexa	Brand name: Citalopram
Generic name: Paxil	Brand name: Paroxetine
Generic name: Luvox, Luvox CR	Brand name: Fluvoxamine
Generic name: Prozac	Brand name: Fluoxetine

Uses: Depression, anxiety, stress, phobias, OCD

Side effects: drowsiness, nausea, lower back or side pain, constipation or diarrhea, headache, dry mouth, tiredness, insomnia

SNRI's

| Generic name: Cymbalta | Brand name: Duloxetine |
| Generic name: Effexor | Brand name: Venlafaxine |

Uses: Anxiety, Depression

Side effects: nausea, dry mouth, increased sweating, appetite loss, insomnia, drowsiness, fatigue, headache

Generic name: Trazodone   Brand name: Oleptro

Uses: Depression, anxiety, insomnia

Side effects: Dry mouth, drowsiness, headache

Generic name: Valproic Acid   Brand name: Depakote, Depakene, Stavzor

Uses: Headache/ migraine prevention, bipolar disorder

Side effects: Indigestion, nausea, vomiting, diarrhea

TOPICAL RETINOIDS

Generic name: Tazarotene	Brand name: Avage, Fabior, Tazorac
Generic name: Tretinoin	Brand name: Avita, Renova, Retin-A
Generic name: Adapalene	Brand name: Differin, Epiduo

Uses: Acne

Side effects: Irritation, redness, dryness, itching, burning

Notes: These work by unclogging the pores so an antibiotic can come in and clear up the infection.

Generic name: Zaleplon   Brand name: Sonata

Uses: Short term insomnia

Side effects: Dizziness, headache, nausea

Generic name: Zolpidem   Brand name: Ambien, Ambien CR, Edluar
Uses: Insomnia
Side effects: Headache, dizziness, diarrhea, nausea

Keeping a medication diary or log will help you to see if your symptoms are improving or getting worse. One or two months are a good time frame to accurately judge what effects the medications or supplements will have on your body. Look below for a sample log to use as an example to make your own or make copies of.

Day	Date	Time	Dose	Name	Side Effects	Conditions taken
Monday	2/22/14	4:00pm	2pills	Vitex	None	With dinner

Medication Lingo

AC- Before meals	Ad Lib- As desired	Bid -twice a day
C- with	et- and	gtt- drops
h/hr- hour	hs -at bedtime	M -mix
od- right eye	os- left eye	ud- as directed
pc- after meals	po -by mouth	prn- as needed
q- each	qd -each day	q hr- each hour
qid -four times daily	s -without	ss- one half
stat -at once	tid- three times a day	

CHAPTER 4- THE IMPORTANCE OF THE RIGHT DOCTOR

There is an old saying that goes "It takes a village to raise a child". Unfortunately, sometimes it takes a village to create one as well. You know what I am talking about. There is a whole slew of different doctors and appointments we have to go to just attempting to get everything in our body to line up the way it is supposed to be. It's nothing to be ashamed of or embarrassed about. Life happens to the best of us.

Here are some important titles that help:

- Dietician
- Nutritionist
- Counselor
- Dermatologist
- Reproductive endocrinologist
- Ob/gyn
- Family practitioner
- Psychiatrist
- Psychologist
- Therapist
- Social worker

➤ Ob/gyn: Their job is to treat the problems that involve the female reproductive system. They also care for women during pregnancy and deliver babies.

➤ Reproductive endocrinologist: Their job is to treat women who suffer from infertility. They will usually see a woman until she is between 8 to 10 weeks pregnant.

➤ Dermatologist: Treats problems of the skin.

➤ Nutritionist: Helps with weight loss and dieting by creating a nutrition plan.

➤ Psychiatrist: They have obtained a M.D. and are able to prescribe medication.

➤ Family Practitioner: Often times your HMO will require that you see a family practitioner before a specialist.

DIAGNOSE YOUR DOCTOR

What are FOUR things you enjoy the MOST about your doctor?

1_____

_____

2_____

_____

3_____

_____

4_____

_____

What are FOUR things you absolutely DON'T enjoy about your doctor?

1_____

_____

2_____

_____

3_____

_____

4_____

_____

How do you envision the PERFECT doctor for YOU?

_____

_____

What is your current doctor like?

_____

_____

What is their experience with PCOS, availability, location, and credentials like?

_____

_____

How well does what you WANT and what you HAVE match up?

_____

_____

It is so important to find a doctor you like. Let's face it; all doctors were not created equally. You need someone you can communicate openly and honestly with. There are many resources available to you to help you locate the best physician for your needs. The best two ways are to call a physician referral line or to ask your friends and family about doctors they like. Word of mouth counts for a lot.

Once you have a place or two in mind that you're interested in, it's beneficial to call the facility and ask a few questions. You'll want to know things like:

- Is this an individual practice? If so what happens when/if that doctor is unavailable
- Is this a group practice? If so can you pick your preferred doctor or do they pick for you
- What hospital is the doctor affiliated with?
- What are the doctor's credentials and business history?
- Does the doctor accept your insurance? If not, what are the fees? Will they require you to pay up front or will you be billed?
- How do they handle emergencies especially after hours?
- What if you have a question, how is it handled? Can you email/call? How soon are they followed up?
- Have they treated people with your condition before?

If the doctor you visit doesn't seem to be a good fit for you, it's okay to move on and find someone more similar to what you're looking for. The bottom line is regardless of what that choice may end up being, the choice is yours. They work for you. You should never feel pressured to undergo or pass up on anything by your doctor.

Before your appointment, gather everything you will need including your insurance card. It is helpful to make a list of questions that you have for the doctor. Don't be afraid to ask your doctor to repeat anything that you didn't fully understand. Maintain an active role in your treatment plan by asking questions.

When you arrive at your first appointment, expect a full workup to be done. It doesn't always happen that way but be prepared just in case. Your physician will ask questions about your last menstrual period (LMP), any changes in weight and the symptoms you are experiencing. They will do a physical exam to get your blood pressure, height, weight and possibly waist size. All that will help them to track your BMI. They may do a pelvic exam and or an ultrasound which will allow your physician to see your ovaries and to check the number of cysts as well as the size of your ovaries. You might also get your blood drawn to check your current hormone levels.

FUN FACT

<u>Hormone is a Greek work that means to set in motion</u>

Your initial meeting should give you an idea of your compatibility. We all have something different that we want or need from our doctor. Finding the right one is crucial.

It's common to have some questions to ask your physician during your appointment. There is nothing wrong with that, they are there to help. Make a list before your appointment and pick the three that are most important to you to ask first. You may have time for more but if not, at least those are taken care of.

You want a doctor who is able to really listen to your problems. You want someone who keeps up to date on current information regarding PCOS, treatments and symptoms. You want someone who can be empathetic to your symptoms and approach them compassionately. Most importantly, you want someone who takes the time to address your concerns.

Keep in mind your physician has other patients that need to be seen as well. They deserve as much attention as you so don't be upset if you don't get everything answered in that appointment. Your physician is not blowing you off; they have a schedule to keep to be fair to all of their patients. If you were not able to cover all of your questions, ask them if you can leave the list with them. This way they can review it when they have some free time and email or call you with the answers at their convenience. Alternatively the physician might be able to delegate questions to the nurse to answer for you.

Any doctor you decide upon needs you to be 100% honest and upfront with them, especially regarding anything you are putting into your body or any new symptoms you are experiencing. Certain things can interact with each other and cause some not so great reactions. It is crucial to inform your physician of everything, even alternative treatments and supplements. It is not their job to like it, just know about it. Most importantly, regardless of what your physician says, you can and should get a second opinion.

While we are on the subject of doctors, let's discuss insurance companies. They can certainly be a hassle, can't they?

Here are some tips to help make your experience a little more enjoyable.

- ✓ Always write down dates, times and names of who you speak to and or write to with title and department
- ✓ If you do mail anything, sending it by certified mail is best. This requires a signature as receipt of its arrival
- ✓ Make copies of any and everything you send or get from your insurance company
- ✓ If anything doesn't look right on a bill or if a claim was denied, always call immediately to see what happened. Never agree to something that you are not completely comfortable with. You have the right to file an appeal if the issue is not resolved the way it should be
- ✓ Be sure to check over your insurance policy really well to see what is covered. You should never be under the assumption something will be covered. You need to verify it to be safe.

A few key words to look out for are: alternative care, maternity/reproductive, mental health, acupressure, prescriptions, homeopathic, herbal, acupuncture, chiropractor and x-ray/ labs

Mandated infertility coverage:

Some states have mandated insurance coverage. They are either mandated to cover or mandated to offer. Mandated to cover means health insurance companies are required to provide infertility coverage as a benefit included in each health insurance policy. While they are mandated to cover, they don't all cover to the same extent. Be sure to verify what is covered and up to what amount.

Mandated to offer, on the other hand means health insurance companies have to have infertility coverage in health insurance policies available to be purchased. Even if your insurance company is mandated to offer, some treatments may still be covered in your policy. As of 2015, the following states are mandated to cover:

- Arkansas
- California

- Connecticut
- Illinois
- Maryland
- Hawaii
- Montana
- New jersey
- Massachusetts
- Louisiana
- New York
- Ohio
- Texas
- Rhode island
- West Virginia

CHAPTER 5- BLOOD WORK

As we know, PCOS is a hormonal imbalance. There are many different hormones in your body that can be affected and get out of balance.

- Cortisol
- Estrogen
- Progesterone
- Androgens

Let's assume that we all have regular cycles and that our glorious aunt flow arrives when she is supposed to every month. When she arrives, a smoke signal of sorts goes out to the pituitary gland from the hypothalamus. Basically it is telling the pituitary gland to begin secreting FSH. The FSH makes its way to your ovaries and stimulates the follicles to begin growing. Each one of these follicles contains an egg and estrogen. When the estrogen level gets high enough, another smoke signal goes out for LH to be released. This is how the process of ovulation begins.

Most cycles run between 21 to 35 days with ovulation typically occurring on day 14. With PCOS, we know our cycle can be completely off course with what it should be doing. Let's take a look at what a "normal" period is like.

Cycle day 1: This is the first day bleeding begins. LH & FSH are released by the pituitary gland and the FSH signals follicles to grow.

Cycle day 7: A bunch of small follicles is growing. There is one larger follicle known as the dominant follicle. Inhibin is being produced.

Cycle day 10: All the smaller follicles begin to disappear and FSH levels start dropping.

Cycle day 13: The one dominant follicle keeps growing and should be getting close to 20mm in diameter. Your LH surges telling ovulation it is now time to start.

Cycle day 14: Ovulation occurs 24-36 hours after LH surge.

Cycle day 21: if you didn't get pregnant, your progesterone level drops and your corpus luteum shrinks.

By the time you have made your entrance in this world, you had all the eggs that you will ever have for your whole life. A rough estimate of this number is approximately 2 million. By the time menstruation begins, it has dropped to half a million or so. You'll only ovulate between 350-500 eggs throughout your life. Your ovarian reserve can be checked to tell approximately how many eggs you have left. The important thing to remember is just because you have periods does not mean your ovary is releasing an egg. As a matter of fact, if you have higher levels of male hormones like testosterone, it can prevent the dominant follicle from being released.

Here's the low down on progesterone.

Having a period does more good for your body than you probably realize. Progesterone is what causes your lining to shed and start a period. If you don't have period, your doctor will more than likely prescribe you a medication such as provera which is progesterone. If your body doesn't make enough progesterone, you won't have a period. Having a period is important because it allows your endometrium to grow, since that is the lining that sheds. It the endometrium is unable to shed, the risk of cancer grows. In fact, endometrial cancer is more often found in women who are obese, have high blood pressure and diabetes. It is also associated with irregular menstrual cycles, inconsistent ovulation and infertility. Having a period at least once every three months helps to shed that lining and reduce the risk of cancer.

Another highly common hormonal imbalance among women is low progesterone levels. It can be caused by aging, stress, high prolactin levels and little to no ovulation. Aging goes hand in hand with ovulation problems. Ovulation helps with production of progesterone. As you get older, you ovulate less. If your progesterone level is low, you may be prescribed medication to raise it. You should obtain a progesterone reading on cycle day 21, with levels being between 15 to 25 ng/mL. A few symptoms are:

- Infertility

- Bloating

- Heavy periods

- Painful periods

- First trimester miscarriage

- Painful breasts

- Irregular menstrual cycles

- Ovarian cysts

A high cortisol level is one of the most common hormonal imbalances that affect women. As a point of reference, you want your cortisol levels to fall between 10 to 15 mcg/dL. The best time to have your blood tested for a cortisol reading is in the morning, usually before 10:00am. Elevated cortisol can cause many problems that you may not even attribute to it, such as:

- Insomnia or trouble staying asleep

- Anxiety

- Decreased fertility

- Irritability

- Memory fog or feeling distracted

- High blood pressure

- Irregular menstrual cycles

- High blood sugar or blood sugar instability

- Indigestion

Excess androgens are probably the biggest problem women with PCOS face. It is the most common endocrine problem that causes infertility in women. Some symptoms of increased androgen levels are:

- Acne

- Skin tags

- Depression

- Anxiety

- Ovarian cysts

- Irregular menstrual cycles

- Hirsutism

- Alopecia

- PCOS

- Infertility

Low estrogen stimulates appetite and basically tells you that you're hungry and need food. Thus, the lower your estrogen is, the hungrier you'll be. It also gives you hot flashes, insomnia and night sweats. Here are some solutions:

- Avoid coffee and caffeine
- Cut out gluten
- Acupuncture
- Add flaxseed and whole soy to your diet
- Limit exercise
- Supplement with Valerian, Magnesium, Vitamin E and Maca

COMMON BLOOD TESTS

- FSH- This test is done on day 3 of your cycle. Too low of FSH levels could indicate declining fertility or approaching menopause.
- Estradiol (aka E2) - This test is done on day 3 of your cycle. It may possibly be redone mid-luteal phase. Estradiol is responsible for creating fertile quality cervical fluid. It stimulates egg and endometrial maturation for the implantation of a fertilized egg.

- Inhibin B- This test is done on day 3 of your cycle. It can predict ovarian reserve (egg quality and quantity) Inhibin-B is a protein hormone. It inhibits FSH.
- Prolactin- This test can be done on any day of your cycle. Prolactin not only stimulates breast milk production, it also stops production of estrogen from the ovaries. Prolactin levels are usually lowest in the morning so levels should be checked before 11:00am. It is made by the anterior pituitary and has numerous things that can raise its levels. Things such as stress, under active thyroid, pituitary adenoma (lump), antidepressants, anti-nausea medication. Bromocriptine and Cabergoline are medications that lower prolactin levels.
- DHEAS- This test can be done on any day of your cycle. It produces issues similar to those of androgens.
- LH- This test is done close to ovulation. When LH surges, it triggers ovulation. It normally spikes about 24-36 hours before you ovulate.
- Progesterone- This test is done mid-luteal phase around cycle day 21. Progesterone is needed to sustain pregnancy early on as well as to sustain uterine lining.
- TSH- TSH helps regulate body hormones and stimulates thyroxine production.
- Testosterone- It's used to help rule out tumors specifically adrenal and ovarian, as the reason behind excessive androgen levels. It is needed to produce estrogen.
- SHBG (Sex hormone binding globulin)- Measures your SHBG levels.
- 17-Hydroxyprogesterone- A test done to check your adrenal glands to rule out CAH which is congenital adrenal hyperplasia. CAH means your adrenal glands don't produce enough cortisol resulting in overproduction of androgens.

There are many diagnostic tests that your doctor may perform to give them a better look at your insides. These tests will allow them to see if any surgeries need to be completed, among other things.

- HSG (Hysterosalpingography): This is a test that allows the physician to see if your fallopian tubes are open or blocked. The test involves being injected through your cervix with a contrast medium, which is a dye that contains iodine. Be sure to let the nurse know if you are allergic to shellfish. The dye branches out to your uterus and your fallopian tubes. The physician then does an x-ray to see if there are any blockages. The dye shows up white on the x-ray. ***FUN FACT*** Back in the 4th century BC, the Greeks actually believed the uterus was not attached to anything and it just wandered around inside the body causing hysteria. This is where the prefix "hyster" comes from.
- Hysteroscopy: During this procedure your uterus is filled with a gas through your cervix. Next your physician will insert a hysteroscope into your uterus. A hysteroscope is a

small telescope with a light on it, the inside is hollow which enables the physician to pass various instruments through it should they see any growths or abnormalities of your uterus. This allows for immediate corrections. You are typically given a local or general anesthetic.

✧ Laparoscopy: A laparoscope is much like a hysteroscope, a small telescope with a light. During a laparoscopy the physician makes a small cut around or even possibly in your belly button. Through this cut, the laparoscope is inserted into your abdominal cavity, which is filled with a gas. After which a colored dye is injected into your fallopian tubes and uterus. You will be given a general anesthetic. Diathermy and drilling can be done during a laparoscopy if needed.

✧ Ovarian Drilling: A small incision is made close to your belly button through which a small tool is inserted into your stomach. This tool is similar to a telescope with a light at the end. Your ovary is punctured with a needle that is carries electricity. This procedure may increase your chance of ovulation however it may only be a temporary fix. It may also lower androgen levels; however you may develop scar tissue on the ovary.

Ways to check for ovulation:

~ Purchase a monitor:
  - Clearblue easy fertility monitor- You will purchase the monitor and sticks separately. Pricing and ordering can be done on their website; www.clearblueeasy.com. The Clearblue monitor works by determing the peak phase of your cycle based off of the LH and estrogen levels in your urine. The Clearblue monitor typically runs close to the $200 mark.
  - OV watch fertility predictor- The watch and sensors are purchased separately. You can view their website at www.ovwatch.com. You wear the watch and it measures ions on your skin which allow it to predict a fertile window.
  - Ovacue fertility monitor- The Ovacue monitor measures electrolyte levels in your spit to tell you when you're approaching ovulation. It can usually tell you within 7 days of ovulation. You can view their website at www.ovacue.com. The Ovacue monitor typically runs close to the $300 mark.
  - Ferning tests- This type of ovulation prediction offers a special microscope that you view saliva through. When you're getting ready to ovulate, the saliva on the lens will form a "ferning" pattern. An example of a ferning test is Fertile- Focus.
~ Purchase a BBT: BBT stands for Basal Body Thermometer. Every morning when you wake up, before you do anything else you will take your temperature and chart it. When your cycle begins, your temperature is lower. When you ovulate, it rises and will stay up higher until right before your next cycle begins.

~ Check your CM: Cervical Mucus will change before you ovulate, both in quality and quantity. It will stay like that through ovulation. EWCM is what you're looking for. That is egg white cervical mucus. It should be able to stretch between your fingers which is a German word known as "spinnbarkeit".

~ Purchase disposable OPK.

PCOS raises LH levels higher than other women; therefor ovulation tests that work based off of LH levels can be less accurate resulting in false positives.

CHAPTER 6 – ADDITIONAL WAYS TO BETTER HEALTH

-Stop smoking

-Weight Loss

-Exercise

If you smoke, stop! Seriously, there are so many health risks that come from smoking. Couple that with the risks we are already facing by just having PCOS. If you are trying to conceive, now is the time to quit. Clear your mind of negative thoughts regarding "how hard" it may be or the possibility of failure.

Much like cocaine, nicotine is very addictive. As a matter of fact, nicotine reaches your brain as quickly as TEN seconds after being inhaled!

Create a plan to help you quit

» The first step in quitting is deciding you're ready and willing to quit!

» Make a list of all the reasons you have to quit (Health, financial, kids, your job, etc). Whatever the reasons may be, keep a copy of this list in different places so you can always review it daily.

» Set a quit date.

MY QUIT DATE IS: _____

» Begin conditioning yourself for the big change to occur. This includes resting and exercising more, increasing your fluids, and reducing your consumption.

» Begin tracking your triggers (situations, places, people, feelings) so you can avoid them.

» Switch your brand of cigarette to something you prefer much less.

» Collect all smoking paraphernalia in a box (lighters, ashtrays, etc) and trash it.

» Find a support system that you can lean on during tough times such as friends and family.

» Set rules for this process such as no smoking in the house or your car. Tell friends and family not to offer you cigarettes and say no if you ask.

» Begin spending more time in places where smoking is prohibited.

» Find alternatives to tobacco such as candy, toothpicks, gum, or lollipops.

» Prepare yourself for situations that are stressful. Have your support system to fall back on. Try a squeeze ball, take a short walk, read a book or even a hot shower.

» On your quit date, trash all your remaining tobacco products.

» Visit the dentist for a good teeth cleaning to start your new life with a new mouth.

Fun Fact

Did you know smoking a pack a day at $5.00 per pack for one year equals out to approximately $1825.00!

Fun Fact

More than 440 thousand people die yearly from tobacco related illnesses

If you are worried about the urge to smoke while quitting, there are medications available to help. Chantix (Varenicline) and Zyban (Bupropion) are a few.

ASRM says 13% of female infertility results from smoking cigarettes. It can also bring on early menopause. In men it can lower sperm count, make sperm slow and increase the percentage of abnormal sperm. (4)

Most withdrawal symptoms can be felt just a few short hours after you finish your last cigarette. Common withdrawal symptoms are:

o Depression Cravings Mood swings Nervousness Insomnia Headaches
o Tiredness Feeling dizzy Eating more Irritability Feeling restless Poor concentration

These symptoms can last anywhere from a couple days to a couple weeks. Hypnosis and acupuncture have been said to help ease the symptoms of withdrawal. Keep in mind that weight gain may be a very real possibility after quitting. This is partly due to nicotine suppressing your appetite and speeding up your system. Don't be discouraged by this. Low fat food choices and other healthy snack replacements including more water and exercise can help keep gaining to a minimum. Sometimes we have to put food in our mouth to keep the smoking urges at bay. Try sunflower seeds, sugarless gum, ice, carrot or celery sticks, air popped popcorn, low fat cottage cheese or lemon drops.

STOP SMOKING PLAN

    1.) Why is quitting important to me?

_____

_____

    2.) What is an ideal quit date?

_____

_____

    3.) What are steps I can take to ensure my success?

_____

_____

    4.) Support team

Names: Numbers:

_____

_____

_____

_____

Let's talk about healthy eating specifically the glycemic index and what it can do for you. If you haven't heard of it, allow me to explain. G.I. stands Glycemic Index. The foods you eat are ranked from 1 to 100 based upon how they interfere with our glucose levels. The foods that are ranked closer to 100 raise glucose levels faster than food ranked closer to 1.

Low G.I. = 55 or less

Medium G.I. = 56 to 69

High G.I. = 70 or more

Carrots	35	Tomato Soup	38
Cheerios	75	Apple	38
Raisins	64	Lowfat yogurt	33
Orange	44	Lima Beans	31
Peach	42	Grapefruit	25
Pineapple	66	Cantaloupe	65
Rice Cakes	77	White Bread	71
Bananas	54	Kiwi	53
Pears	37	Grapes	46
Lentils	29	Cherries	22

If you're able to stick to a low G.I. diet, your glucose levels will remain lower. In turn, this lowers the need for your body to make more insulin. The lower the G.I. number of the food, the slower it is digested. This helps you to feel fuller much longer. Fiber also helps lower the G.I. number of foods. Before low or high G.I. foods came to be, carbohydrates were classified only as simple or complex. That represents the structure of their chemical nature.

Complex carbs are digested slowly which results in a smaller rise in glucose levels compared to simple carbs that are digested fast causing a rapid rise.

A low G.I. diet is much more than a diet. It really is a way of life. It's important to insulin resistant people for many reasons.

-    When you eat foods that are higher on the glycemic index list, your pancreas has a high amount of insulin that it must produce.

- Eating foods that are lower on the glycemic index list help keep your insulin levels lower which then allows your body to burn fat and raises your metabolic rate. If your insulin level was high, your body would be burning carbohydrates and not fat.
- Foods that have a lower glycemic index number are healthy options carbohydrate wise and they also are high in fiber. Fiber is excellent for your body. Not only does It make you feel fuller faster and longer, it also helps to keep your bowels regular in the bathroom.
- Low G.I. foods help to keep our immune system healthy which in turn means less allergies and milder symptoms. This is because low G.I. foods mean low insulin levels. Low insulin levels encourage our immune systems to function better.

Eating foods that are higher on the glycemic index list causes our glucose levels to spike and then drop rather quickly. This happens partly because these foods bring about a rush of sugar into our blood stream. The pancreas doesn't know what to do and does the best thing it can which is release insulin; however it releases too much insulin. The glucose level drops and cortisol is released which is why we feel hungry again so quickly after eating.

You can spot a low G.I. food by looking for the Glycemic Index symbol. It is a circle with a large G inside of it. More information can be found at www.GIsymbol.com

Be sure to still keep an eye on your caloric intake even while on a low G.I. plan. Calories can hinder weight loss and add up very fast.

There are so many low G.I. foods that are excellent replacements.

- ✓ Instead of the whole egg, eat only egg whites
- ✓ Switch to skim milk if you don't already drink it
- ✓ Eat whole wheat grains like bread and pasta
- ✓ Get fat free food like cottage cheese, salad dressing and mayonnaise
- ✓ Load up on fruits: oranges, grapes, peaches, grapefruit, cherries and more
- ✓ You can never go wrong with vegetables! Bell peppers, peas, zucchini, lettuce, etc.

I highly recommend reading a book called *The Glycemic Index Diet* by Rick Gallop. He has ingeniously created a "traffic light" layout throughout his book. This enables the reader to effortlessly glide through to see what is not healthy, what is semi- healthy and what is the healthiest according to the glycemic index. He also lists multiple G.I. friendly recipes to try.

Now that we know a little bit about the glycemic index, let's talk about the glycemic load (G.L.). It's a little different from the G.I. as it tells us the amount of carbs in foods whereas the glycemic index refers to how quickly that particular food will affect our glucose level.

High G.L. → GL of 20 and up

Medium G.L. → GL of 11-19

Low G.L. → GL of 10 and under

Each day you should plan to take in a G.L. of 60-75. Ideally, you'll want this amount spaced out throughout the entire day.

BMI CHART

	19	20	21	22	23	24	25	26	27
5'3"	107	113	118	124	130	135	141	146	152
5'4"	110	116	122	128	134	140	145	151	157
5'5"	114	120	126	132	138	144	150	156	162
5'6"	118	124	130	136	142	148	155	161	167

Interpret BMI Chart:

Underweight: less than 18.5

Normal: 18.5-24.9

Overweight: 25-29.9

Obese: 30 or more

One pound is equal to 3600 calories. With that being said, cutting back 500 calories per day will equate to 3500 calories per week which is pretty close to one pound. Most of us probably consume close to 1200 and 1500 calories per day. Realistically a 500 calorie reduction isn't impossible. You shouldn't cut out more than that because your metabolic rate will slow down and hinder your weight loss doing more harm than good.

Here are some tips:

~ Avoid or limit alcohol. Just a gentle reminder that alcohol DOES contain carbs and calories!
~ Space carbs throughout the day to avoid sugar spikes in one meal
~ Eat 40% carbs, pick low G.I. Carbs

~ Add Omega-3 Fatty Acids to your diet. They may help to improve glucose levels and lower cholesterol

~ Increase daily fiber intake. There is a seed very high in fiber called Psyllium. You can purchase it at health food stores in powdered form and mix it into a glass of water. Psyllium helps to slow the digestion of carbohydrates

~ Always combine carbs with a protein or a fat, never eat it alone

~ Eat regular meals that are fairly spaced out during the day

~ Drink at least eight 8 ounce glasses of water daily

~ Limit sodium intake

~ Avoid caffeine as much as possible. Caffeine decreases fertility levels and increases your risk of miscarriage.

~ When you drink water that is extra cold your body will burn more calories. This happens because our body needs to work harder to attempt to counteract the waters temperature.

~ Don't be fooled by the fancy words on food labels. When you see "ose" at the end of the word, it is sugar! For instance, dextrose and fructose are fruit sugar while sucrose is table sugar

A food journal is an excellent way to track what you're eating and help you to be accountable for it.

Check out www.mayoclinic.com or www.webmd.com to use their online calorie counter.

To be successful in controlling your weight issues, it is not only about being able to lose the weight. You need to also be able to keep the weight off. To do that, you need to set goals for yourself that are SMART.

SMART stands for Specific, Measurable, Achievable, Realistic and Time specific.

Example: I currently weight 195 pounds. I want to be down to 175 pounds in 5 months. I can achieve this by losing 4 pounds a month for 5 months which is 1 pound a week.

Specific → down to 175 pounds

Measurable → 1 pound a week

Time specific → 5 months

Weigh yourself once or twice a week but no more than that.

Monounsaturated fats are incredibly beneficial to us and they can help us to lose weight. They reduce our insulin resistance, lower LDL levels and support our immune system. You can find them in foods like olives, avocados, almonds, hazelnuts, brazil nuts, sesame seeds, cashews, peanuts, oil and peanut oil to name a few. Monounsaturated fats contain very little to no carbs and are also considered low G.I. foods.

Have you heard of xenoestrogents? They come from things like herbicides and pesticides. You can find them on the skin of chickens, by microwaving food in plastic containers and on fruits and vegetables that aren't organically grown. They can stimulate certain health problems like breast cancer, ovarian cysts and menstrual irregularities.

Metabolism:

I'm sure you've heard someone say that people with fast metabolisms can eat anything and stay skinny. Here is the problem: the more body fat you have, the slower your metabolism is. The slower your metabolism is, the harder it is to lose weight. See the pattern there?

Ways to boost your metabolism:

- Eat spicy peppers in your meals
- Don't overeat
- Limit or avoid caffeine
- Get an adequate amount of sleep
- Increase your muscle mass by strength training

Resistance training is any exercise that makes your muscles work against a resistance. It is crucial to strengthen muscles, achieve and maintain good posture and tone your body. By building a little leaner muscle mass; you increase your metabolic rate.

Your basal metabolic rate, or BMR, is something you might hear a lot of. Harris - Benedict formula is used to calculate your BMR. Your BMR is the rate that your body burns calories while it is at rest. It accounts for approximately 60% to 75% of the calories you burn daily by simply living.

Formula:

1. Multiply weight in pounds by 4.3:_____
2. Multiply height in inches by 4.7:_____
3. Multiply age in years by 4.7:_____
4. Add lines 1 and 2, then subtract line 3:_____
5. Add 655 to line 4= Your BMR

H2O

The importance of water cannot be over stated. Two thirds of our body is in fact, water. This is why it is so crucial to keep our supply refreshed often.

Water has so many benefits, such as:

- Helping your kidney and liver to function properly and flush out toxins

- Reducing headaches

- More energy

- Helps digestive system function properly

- Helps immune system function more efficiently

- You burn more fat

- Joints are more lubricated

A good number to aim for is 6-8 eight ounce glasses of water every day.

Here's a tip: by the time your brain tells you that you're thirsty, you have already reached a point of mild dehydration. Being dehydrated can increase swelling in our face, ankles and legs. Not only that but it can also cause us to have headaches and become highly irritable.

Ever wonder why you constantly wake up in the middle of the night? Your body is talking to you. 1-3 am is the peak time when your liver is "awake".

Want to improve the health of your heart and lungs? I know you do, so what are you waiting for, go exercise!

It is recommended you work out for 5 to 7 days per week for 30 minutes of moderate intensity each day.

If your goal is to lose weight, try increasing that to 5 days per week for 60 minutes each day or 7 days per week for 40 minutes each day.

There is an unlimited supply of exercise options available for you, even things you may not even think about, like chewing sugar free gum. That burns calories and increases the flow of blood to your brain which in turn makes you feel more alert.

If you'd rather skip the routines, try these ideas:

- Park at the far end of the lot when you go shopping or at work
- Take the stairs instead of the elevator
- Go into the restaurant instead of going through the drive thru

Exercise does so much good for our bodies. It helps to raise our SHBG and reduce our insulin resistance, because the higher our SHBG levels are, the lower our testosterone levels are.

Do you currently have an exercise routine that works for you? Here are some questions to consider if you don't.

1.) What type of exercises are your favorites? (jumping jacks, running, crunches, squats, etc)
2.) When is the best time for you to do them? (After kids are in bed, before work, etc)
3.) Where are you able to do them? (Basement, yard, park, bedroom, gym, etc)
4.) Do you face any obstacles? (no babysitter, no room, no equipment)
5.) How can you persevere?
6.) What is your current weight?
7.) What is your height?
8.) What is your BMI?
9.) What is your ideal healthy weight according to a healthy BMI of 19-24?

Take a look at the following chart to see how many approximate calories are burned per activity per hour. Again these are just approximate values and vary greatly based upon intensity involved.

Activity	If you're 130lbs	If you're 160lbs	If you're 200lbs
Low impact aerobics	172	211	264
Moderate stationary bicycling	218	269	336
Moderate stair step machine	187	230	288
Basketball	250	307	384

Bicycling 12-13.9mph	250	307	384
Frisbee	94	115	144
Horseback riding	125	154	192
Ice skating	218	269	336
Martial arts	312	384	480
Rope jumping	312	384	480
Running 5mph	250	307	384
Softball	156	192	240
Swimming	187	230	288
Tennis	218	269	336
Volleyball	94	115	144
Walking 3.5mph	125	154	192
Walking 4mph	140	173	216
Walking 4.5mph	156	192	240
Gardening	140	173	216
Housecleaning	109	134	168
Mowing lawn push mower	172	211	264
Walking snow blower	140	173	216
Raking lawn	125	154	192
Sex	47	58	72
Shoveling snow by hand	187	230	288

As you can see there are so many benefits to exercise.

- ✓ Endorphins are released
- ✓ Helps balance estrogen and testosterone
- ✓ Boosts metabolism
- ✓ Heart works better
- ✓ Muscles and bones become stronger
- ✓ Energy levels are raised
- ✓ Body fats reduced
- ✓ Stress is reduced
- ✓ Gain flexibility
- ✓ Get in shape
- ✓ Gain strength
- ✓ Muscles are more defined
- ✓ Increases confidence level
- ✓ Promotes weight loss
- ✓ Reduces body pain

- ✓ Raises HDL
- ✓ Lowers blood pressure
- ✓ Reduces cardiovascular disease risk

Before you set out to exercise here are a few tips:

- Always make sure to warm up before
- Always make sure to cool down after
- Don't exercise after a big meal
- Drink a lot of water
- Do the same amount of exercises on each side of your body
- Don't overdo it or ignore your body's signals

Build muscles up with strength training. Even at rest bigger muscles burn more calories. Strength training also helps strengthen your bones.

Here are some strength training exercises to try: Fitness balls, power yoga, push-ups, sit ups, resistance bands, pull ups, climbing, and free weights (dumbbells)

Cardiovascular exercise can lower high blood pressure. It enables your heart to pump better. This relaxes blood vessels to lower blood pressure.

Aerobic exercises include walking, dance, step class, cycling, swimming, jogging, running, kickboxing, stair climbing

If you're having trouble understanding intensity levels while exercising, here's a tip:

- Low intensity means the ability to carry on a conversation
- Moderate intensity means you can carry on a conversation however it isn't easy
- Vigorous intensity means there is no ability to have a conversation

Intensity levels should be built up over time. Always start slow and small. Do not try to do too much until your body has adjusted to it.

Set a goal of a heart rate that is about 50%-70% of your max heart rate. Use the following calculation:

Take your age and subtract it from 220. The number you get is your max heart rate beats per minute. As an example: if you're 27 years old, 220-27= 193

Multiple your result by 0.5 to get the lower number of your heart rate range. Multiply by 0.7 to get the upper number of your heart rate range. These two numbers are the range you want your heart rate in during levels of moderate intensity.

193x0.5= 96.5 and 193x0.7= 135   the heart rate range for the example is 96.5 - 135

If you would much rather try for weight loss surgery, here are a few of the options available to you.

- Small bowel bypass- After a major weight loss surgery like this, vitamin and mineral supplements usually need to be taken for the rest of your life. During this procedure, a smaller stomach pouch is made from the original stomach. This new smaller stomach usually holds around 1 -2 fluid ounces.
- Gastric Band (Lap band/ Laparoscopic Gastric Banding) - This surgery involves removing a portion of your stomach to reduce the size of it.
- Gastric Balloon – No surgery is needed to obtain a gastric balloon.

Be sure to contact your insurance company prior to any weight loss surgery. You'll want to verify you are covered for the procedure and how much you'll need to pay, as well as the process needed for approval.

CHAPTER 7- SUPPORT SYSTEM

Some cysters would prefer to fight the battle in silence and not tell anyone. Others divulge the hairy details to anybody who will listen. Whichever path you decide upon, the choice lies with you and you alone.

What scares you the most about sharing your diagnosis with others?

_____

_____

Which person are you most fearful about telling?

_____

_____

Why?

_____

_____

What do you have to lose by letting "the cat out of the bag?"

_____

_____

What do you have to gain?

_____

_____

We all need support in one way or another. Joining a support group can be a very intimidating decision but you should never be embarrassed about it. When most people think about finding a support group, AA is usually the first thing that comes to mind. You envision a bunch of strangers sitting in a circle. "Hi my name is Tamara and I have PCOS." In unison they all respond " Hi Tamara." That is not exactly an ideal situation nor is it what I'm referring to when I speak of a support group.

A support group can be anything; friends, family, coworkers, etc. Anyone who is ready and willing to lend an ear in your time of need is a "support group member." If you find it difficult to talk to family about PCOS and your experience, there are many excellent groups to join both locally and online.

They are beneficial to join for many reasons. They offer you new information and advice including different ways to manage your symptoms. It also gives you the opportunity to see that there are numerous other women out there going through the same exact thing as you. Some may have it worse, while some don't. We are all pursing different goals in our journey with PCOS.

What if you can't find a group you like? Well, start your own! Here are a few tips to help get you started.

- It is best to start small with a few loyal members. When groups grow too fast it's possible for some members to lose sight of the "support" factor.
- You can ask around to find new members, talk to friends, put an ad in the local newspaper or online, even post fliers on bulletin boards around town.
- Establish a place and time that you'll meet. Decide if they'll be weekly, biweekly or monthly meetings. You want the place that you use for meetings to be private such as a church or other members homes.
- Will you charge a fee for memberships, rental space donations, food, etc?
- Make sure to keep a member log with names and contact information.

There will be times when people around you make your emotions run rampant. That's okay, embrace those feelings. The truth is, nothing is fair about what we have or what we go through. Every day you see women with flawless skin, no acne or excessive hair meanwhile you are practically buying stock in hair removal products. What about those tight toned bodies? No ma'am, nothing about our struggle is fair. Remember this: it is not about what happens to you. It's about how you respond!

Let me share with you some helpful ways to tame those feelings.

1. First and foremost, I want you to understand that it is OKAY to cry. There is no rule saying you cannot break down and fall apart every so often. In fact it is healthy. You need to release the pain, hurt, anger and all those other pent up feelings or they will eat you alive.
2. Embrace the breakdown. Accept that you need it and that by doing so it does NOT make you weak. It makes you stronger because you know what you need to do to keep it

together the rest of the time. You recognize the way you feel which means you can approach them with a clear head.

3. Start writing in a journal. This will allow you to confront feelings you might not have noticed were buried inside of you. It will also help you to learn how to express your feelings in a way that is more appropriate. Instead of lashing out at someone or isolating yourself, write.

4. Talk to yourself, seriously! When you feel your emotions are about to boil over, remind yourself that you CAN handle this. The next time your mother in law asks when you're going to have kids, smile and say to yourself "I'm in control, her words can't hurt me."

5. Most importantly, breathe!

6. Don't blame others.

7. Have sex! Lots of it, without schedules, or planning.

8. Educate yourself about what you are going through and will go through.

With the toll PCOS takes on us physically, mentally and emotionally, it is easy to forget how incredible we are. It is even easier to not believe others when they remind us. Sometimes we have to learn how to love ourselves after our diagnosis. We can become our own worst critic. Try hanging post it notes around your home as daily reminders to stop being so hard on yourself.

You are beautiful!

Weight does not define you!

You are not owned by PCOS

Smile bright

You are strong

You are smart

You are a survivor

Take the time right now and show yourself why you are one rockin' cyster!

I am beautiful because_____
_____

I deserve love because_____

_____

My favorite thing about myself is_____

_____

I'm the best at_____

_____

I AM ONE ROCKIN' CYSTER!

Who do you know or know of that has PCOS?	What do you love about them? (inspiration, uniqueness, confidence)
Victoria Beckham from The Spice Girls	
Jillian Michaels	

Stress-

Stress is something that none of us want to be bothered with. It comes so easy, especially with the daily PCOS dramas. However most of us are completely unaware of the negative toll it has on our bodies.

Inside of our body is a stress hormone, it is called cortisol. When we are under a lot of stress, cortisol causes insulin levels to increase. Since insulin is the hormone responsible for making our bodies store fat, it comes as no surprise that the connection between cortisol and insulin is why we store it all particularly around our midsection. When both hormones are elevated, exercising to lose the belly bulge will achieve little results. Controlling your stress level is important for many reasons, not only because if your cortisol levels stay high too much it can lead to conditions like high blood pressure, cancer, heart disease, diabetes and weight gain. Also, serotonin is "drained" by cortisol.

Serotonin is a neurotransmitter, which means a chemical in your brain. It is mainly responsible for helping you to relax and increasing your mood. That leads us back to the vicious cycle; when you're stressed, you're not happy.

To reduce stress, give some of the following techniques a try:

- » Deep breathing
- » Exercise
- » Laughter
- » Music therapy
- » Prayer
- » Tai Chi or Qigong
- » Visualization
- » Yoga

CHAPTER 8 – ALTERNATIVE MEDICINE

These are methods that are used while not on a traditional medication treatment.

-VITAMINS   -HERBS   -MINERALS

Caution: before starting any new form of alternative medicine, always consult a doctor first. There are many potential pros and cons that should be discussed with a health care professional. Some alternative treatments can interact with others. Be sure to check all labels. Ask if you're ever unsure. Don't assume because the label says natural that it is safe. There are many highly poisonous natural things out there; an example being arsenic. It is always best to ask about alternative treatment combinations rather than assume there will not be an adverse effect from it. If you can't find the right answers, don't use it until you do.

These are not regulated by the Food and Drug Administration. The FDA did, however establish current good manufacturing practice requirements or C.G.M.P's for short. The C.G.M.P requirements state that manufacturers of supplements must report serious side effects to the FDA.

When checking over the label, always read directions for use and dosage recommendations. Verify the bottle is not expired and is properly sealed to ensure its freshness.

RDA's, DRI's and TUIL's and what do they all mean. All these letters may sound like just a bunch of jumbled letters, but there really is more to them than that. When trying to figure out how much of a supplement to take you can refer to the daily percent values listed on the containers. If you'd like more detailed information, you should take a look at one of the aforementioned values.

RDA stands for Recommended Dietary Allowance. They are the minimal amount needed to keep our bodies from developing nutrient deficiencies. Basically what a person who is healthy will need to maintain that level of health.

AI stands for Adequate Intake. They are an approximate nutritional value for a group of healthy people. They're used when a RDA value is not available.

DRI stands for Dietary Reference Intake. Made up of four reference values (RDA, AI, EAR, UL) DRI is a more personalized number for age, pregnancy, etc.

TUIL stands for Tolerable Upper Intake Level. It is sometimes referred to as the U.L (Upper Limit). This is the most of that nutrient our bodies can handle without it being too much. While our RDA for Vitamin D is between 5-10mcg our TUIL is 50mcg.

EAR stands for Estimated Average Requirement. This value represents the level of nutrients that could fulfill the requirements of half of the "healthy" people in a group.

What exactly is a vitamin? To put it plainly, a vitamin is something that is needed for us to live. Vitamins are considered micronutrients. This means that only small amounts are needed for our bodies to work correctly. We have 13 essential vitamins. They're either water soluble or fat soluble. Technically speaking, vitamins are organic substances. Most of them are not produced within our body which is why we need to make sure we get enough either through our diets or via a supplement.

Vitamins A, D, E and K are fat soluble. This means excess amounts are stored inside our body.

Vitamins C and the 8 B vitamins (Biotin, Folate, Niacin, Panthothenic Acid, Riboflavin, Thiamine, B6 & B12) are water soluble, meaning excess amounts are released through our urine.

VITAMINS:

Vitamin A

Fat soluble   RDA 700 mcg/ 4000 IU

AKA Retinol, Retinene, Retinoic Acid, Retinyl Palmitate

Benefits:

- Promotes healthy skin, hair, and mucous membranes
- Possibly speeds up healing time
- Treats disorders of the eye
- Counteracts night blindness
- Maintains health and function of sperm cells, egg cells, placenta and ovaries
- Aids in growth of bones and teeth development
- Maintains normal immune system

Natural Sources

- Hard-boiled egg   Broccoli
- Apricots   Milk
- Cantaloupe   Spinach
- Pumpkin pie   Carrots

Herbs:

- Fennel seed   Hops   Kelp   Lemongrass
- Raspberry leaf   Sage   Yellow dock   Watercress

Symptoms of a deficiency:

- Dry, rough skin   Diarrhea   Insomnia
- Trouble with vision (Night blindness)   Weight loss   Acne   Fatigue

Signs of an overdose:

- Vomiting   Headache   Irritability   Nausea   Abdominal pain

- Dry skin   Fatigue   Vision problems

Facts:

- Measured in United States Pharmacopeia units (USP), International units (IU) and Retinol Equivalents (RE)
- The liver can store up to one years' worth of Vitamin A. This stock can be depleted with illness and infections.
- Antibiotics and laxatives can interfere with the absorption of Vitamin A.

Vitamin B12

Water soluble   RDA 2.4mcg

AKA Cobalamin

Benefits:

- Helps to treat anemia (pernicious)
- May help to boost number of sperm cells in men with abnormal production
- Helps to treat Alzheimer's
- Encourages growth
- Needed to produce myelin (protective sheath around nerves)

Natural sources

- Beef   Eggs
- Oysters   Liverwurst
- Herring   Blue Cheese
- Clams   Sardines
- Flounder   Milk
- Swiss cheese   Mackerel

Herbs:

- Alfalfa   Hops

Symptoms of deficiency:

- Weakness   Confusion   Bruising
- Nausea   Fatigue   Depression   Weight loss

Facts:

- Vitamin C may help to improve the absorption of B12 when taken together
- Not enough B6, calcium or iron can interfere with B12 being absorbed
- Measured in Micrograms (mcg)
- Sublingual is the best route for absorption
- Metformin (Glucophage) is known to deplete B12 levels. Oral contraceptives may also deplete B12 levels

Vitamin B6

Water soluble   RDA 1.3mg-1.6mg

AKA Pyridoxine

Benefits:

- Aids in production of energy
- Lower cholesterol
- Reduce PMS symptoms
- Encourages brain to function normally
- Immune system support
- Regulates metabolism
- Helps stabilize blood glucose levels

Natural sources

- Avocados   Salmon
- Shrimp   Sunflower seeds
- Tuna   Potatoes
- Bananas   Salmon
- Lentils   Soybeans

Symptoms of deficiency:

- Weakness   Insomnia   Acne   Anemia
- Irritability   Nervousness   Confusion   Depression

Signs of an overdose:

- Night restlessness   Numb feet   Twitching

Herbs:

- Alfalfa   Catnip   Oatstraw

Facts:

- Birth control should be taken with a B6 supplement
- Measured in milligrams (mg)

Vitamin C

Water Soluble   RDA 60mg- 75mg

AKA Ascorbic Acid

FUN FACT

Vitamin C deficiency was the cause of scurvy among sailor's centuries ago

Benefits:

- Stimulates cortisone production
- Increases amount of iron absorbed from non-meat sources
- Helps to heal wounds
- Anti-oxidant
- Helps prevent cancer

Natural sources

- Potatoes   Green peppers
- Guava   Cabbage
- Lemons   Strawberries

- Tomatoes   Orange juice
- Brussel sprouts   Oranges
- Spinach   Bananas
- Broccoli

Herbs:

- Alfalfa   Burdock Root   Fennel Seed
- Fenugreek   Parsley   Plantain
- Raspberry Leaf   Yarrow   Yellowdock

Symptoms of deficiency:

- Wounds wont heal normally   Diarrhea
- Anemia   Diminished immune function
- Fatigue   Shortness of breath
- Bleeding gums   Nosebleeds
- Easy bruising   Digestive difficulties

Your supply of Vitamin C can be depleted by a few sources that you might not have even thought about.

- Drinking alcohol
- Tobacco use
- Taking birth control pills
- Using aspirin on a regular basis
- Stress

Facts:

- Lack of Vitamin C can make sperm stick/ clump together called sperm agglutination

Vitamin D

Fat soluble   RDA 200-400 IU

AKA Calciferol

Benefits:

- Strengthens bones and teeth
- Controls calcium absorption

- Helps immune and nervous system function normally

Natural sources

- Salmon   Butter
- Herring   Tuna
- Shrimp   Cod liver oil

Symptoms of deficiency:

- Nervousness   Diarrhea
- Insomnia   Muscle twitches
- Bone weakening

Herbs:

- Alfalfa   Nettle   Parsley

Overdose symptoms:

- Nausea   Anorexia   Headache   Weakness

- Unusual thirst   Vomiting

Facts:

- Measured in International Units (IU) Or Micrograms of Cholecalciferol (mcg)

- Helps to prevent Rickets which is a disease of calcium deprived bones. (Bow legs, knock knees and other bone defects)

Vitamin E

Fat Soluble   RDA 15 mg

AKA Tocopherol

Benefits:

- Anti- blood clotting agent
- Encourages normal formation of red blood cells
- Possibly treats acne
- Reduces pms symptoms

- Nourishes endocrine system

Natural sources

- Almonds
- Sunflower seeds
- Eggs
- Broccoli
- Walnuts
- Canola oil
- Wheat germ

- Brazil nuts
- Seafood
- Asparagus
- Hazelnuts
- Avocados
- Spinach

Symptoms of deficiency:

- Lethargy
- Poor concentration
- Easy bruising

- Dry skin
- Dry hair
- Poor wound healing

- Eczema
- Hot flashes
- Muscle weakness

Herbs:

- Alfalfa
- Flaxseed

- Dandelion
- Raspberry Leaf

- Dong Quai

Facts:

- Cholesterol lowering medications may deplete Vitamin E levels
- Vitamin E may cause blood thinning and should be stopped before surgery
- Vitamin E measurements of 1 IU equals 1 mg
- In order for your body to be able to maintain an appropriate level of Vitamin E, your body requires zinc.

Vitamin K

Fat soluble   RDA 60-65mcg

AKA Phytonadione

Benefits:

- Encourages development and growth
- Aids health of bones
- Helps normal blood clotting
- Promotes healthy kidney function
- Anti-oxidant

Natural sources

- Alfalfa   Brussel sprouts
- Spinach   Coffee beans
- Asparagus   Cabbage
- Cauliflower   Cheddar cheese
- Lettuce   Broccoli
- Turnip green   Oats
- Watercress

Herbs:

- Alfalfa   Green Tea   Nettle   Kelp   Shephards Purse

A Vitamin K deficiency is very rare in adults

FUN FACT

Named after the word 'Koagulation'. In the 1930's a Danish researcher, Henrik Dam noted giving a large amount of cabbage to chicks stopped their bleeding. He identified it was the Vitamin K.

Facts:

- Measured in Micrograms (mcg)

Minerals

What is a mineral?

Much like vitamins, we have 16 essential minerals that fall into two different groups; major and trace.

Unlike vitamins however, minerals are inorganic and most of them can be found inside of our bones. Minerals are needed so our hormones and enzymes can function properly. Approximately 4% of our total body weight is minerals.

As the names imply, major minerals are needed in larger amounts which is usually more than 100 millligrams per day while trace minerals are needed in much smaller amounts. Calcium, magnesium, potassium and sodium are a few major minerals. Examples of trace minerals are iron, manganese, selenium and zinc.

Folic Acid

Water soluble   RDA 400mcg

AKA Folate, Vitamin B9

Benefits:

- Aids in normal development of fetus
- Helps red blood cells form normally
- May help raise sperm counts in men
- Needed to make DNA & RNA

FUN FACT

Birth control pills can lower folate levels

Natural sources

- Asparagus   Beans
- Cabbage   Lentils
- Eggs   Fish
- Soybeans   Avocados
- Beets   Cantaloupe
- Garbanzo beans   Celery
- Sunflower seeds   Bananas

- Brussel sprouts   Wheat germ
- Peas   Orange juice
- Cottage cheese

Symptoms of deficiency:

- Irritability   No energy   Upset stomach
- Paleness   Weakness   Diarrhea   No appetite

Folic Acid deficiency can lead to megaloblastic anemia.

FUN FACT

<u>It was given its name because it was first isolated from green leafy vegetables. Folium means "foliage" or "leaf" in latin.</u>

Facts:

- Alcohol and oral contraceptives may increase need for folate

- Measured in Micrograms (mcg)

Calcium

RDA: 1000mg

Benefits:

- Prevention of osteoporosis
- Strengthens bones and teeth
- Aids in muscle and leg cramp prevention
- Helps normal grown and development occur
- Helps body store and release certain hormones
- Aids in blood pressure reduction

Natural sources

- Almonds   Broccoli
- Cheddar cheese   Yogurt
- Pistachios   Kelp
- Milk   Cottage cheese
- Salmon   Eggs
- Brazil nuts   Turnip greens
- Sardines   Parmesan cheese

Symptoms of deficiency:

- Muscle cramps   Frequent fractures   Loss of height   Insomnia

Herbs:

- Burdock Root   Cayenne   Chamomile   Dandelion   Kelp
- Fennel Seed   Fenugreek Hops   Raspberry Leaf   Yarrow

Facts:

- Calcium should be divided for maximum effectiveness. This is because the body struggles to absorb more than 500 milligrams at a time.

Manganese

RDA 2.5mg-5mg

Benefits:

- Essential in the production of estrogen and progesterone
- Creates healthy nervous system
- Aids in digestion
- Helps energy production
- Helps to control blood sugar

Natural sources

- Blueberries   Buckwheat
- Peanuts   Spinach
- Oatmeal   Peas
- Blackberries   Carrots
- Pecans   Tea
- Whole wheat   Strawberries
- Bran   Hazelnuts
- Seaweed   Avocado
- Thyme   Bananas

Facts:

- Too much can interfere with iron absorption and cause iron deficiency
- Measured in milligrams (mg)

FUN FACT

Manganese is derived from a Greek word meaning magic because of how well it works throughout the body

Iron

RDA 15-18mg

Most common form: Ferrous Sulfate

Benefits:

- Reduces menstrual pain
- Triggers hemoglobin production
- Helps correct iron deficiency problems

Natural sources

- Egg yolk   Lentils
- Mussels   Enriched bread
- Pumpkin seeds   Oysters
- Whole grain   Raisins
- Garbanzo beans   Walnuts
- Peanut butter

Repliva is an iron supplement

Herbs:

- Burdock Root   Catnip   Cayenne   Chamomile   Yellow Dock

- Dandelion   Dong Quai   Fennel Seed Fenugreek

- Raspberry Leaf

Symptoms of deficiency:

- Fatigue   Listlessness   Poor concentration
- Irritability Pale appearance

FUN FACT

In 4000 BC the Persian physician Melampus gave iron supplements to sailors to replenish the iron they lost from bleeding wounds suffered during sea battles.

Potassium

RDA 2000mg

Benefits:

- Helps control blood pressure
- Aids in regulating heartbeat
- Possibly reduce acne
- Required for insulin secretion by pancreas

- Helps keep nervous system healthy

Natural sources:

- Asparagus   Kidney beans
- Milk   Fresh peas
- Fish   Nuts
- Spinach   Parsnips
- Carrots   Bananas
- Avocados   Cantaloupe
- Potatoes   Raisins
- Sardines

Herbs:
- Sage   Skullcap   Hops   Nettle   Plantain   Red Clover

Symptoms of deficiency:

- Weakness   Constipation   Depression
- Heart disturbances   Insomnia   Acne
- Fatigue   Mood changes

Facts:

- Potassium can be depleted by excessive diarrhea or vomiting, excessive intake of alcohol, caffeine, salt, sugar and stress

- A single banana can contain 500 milligrams of potassium

Magnesium

RDA 310mg-400mg

Benefits:

- Helps bones grow
- Lowers risk of diabetes
- Helps to strengthen enamel on teeth

- Helps regulate blood pressure
- Helps regulate sleep cycles / biological clock
- Helps with energy production

Natural sources

- Almonds	Bluefish
- Collards	Halibut
- Shrimp	Cashews
- Dried prunes	Peanuts
- Dandelion greens	Soybeans
- Avocados	Carp
- Herring	Tofu
- Coconut	Dried apricots
- Pumpkin seeds	Spinach
- Bananas	Cod
- Flounder	Dried figs
- Kelp	Dates
- Brazil nuts	Parsley
- Sunflower seeds	Sesame seeds

Herbs:

- Catnip	Cayenne	Chamomile	Dandelion
- Raspberry Leaf	Sage	Yarrow	
- Fenugreek	Fennel Seed	Yellow Dock	

Symptoms of deficiency:

- Muscle contractions	Teeth grinding	Sleep talking	Insomnia
- Confusion	Sleep walking	Night terrors	Skin problems
- Nervousness	Nausea	Irritability	

Facts:
- Magnesium needs increase with stress or illness as well as alcohol
- Measured in Milligrams (mg)
- Magnesium can lower dopamine levels which are a chemical in the brain that helps to regulate moods.

Selenium

RDA 55mcg

Benefits:

- helps to stimulate the immune system
- helps prevent miscarriage and birth defects
- Helps to combat dandruff, eczema and warts
- Anti-oxidant
- Helps to maintain viability of sperm cells

Natural sources:

- Bran   Cabbage
- Milk   Seafood
- Whole grains Broccoli
- Garlic   Mushrooms
- Walnuts   Asparagus
- Brown rice   Liver
- Onions   Brazil nuts
- Eggs

Herbs:

- Burdock Root   Catnip   Chamomile   Cayenne
- Fenugreek   Raspberry Leaf Yarrow   Yellow Dock
- Fennel Seed

Facts:

- Consuming too much selenium can lead to selenosis, which is excessively high levels. Symptoms of selenosis are gastrointestinal disorders, hair loss, irritability, and brittle nails to name a few.

- Selenium deficiency has been linked to cancer and heart disease

Symptoms of deficiency:

- Poor immune function

Zinc

RDA 15-30mg

Benefits:

- Helps fetus grow
- Keeps vitamin A level in blood normal
- Reduces burns and wounds
- Promotes fertility and reproductive development
- Helps combat dandruff
- Helps regulate immune system
- Helps keep eyes healthy
- Helps regulate appetite

Natural sources

- Beef   Egg
- Milk   Sunflower seeds
- Wheat germ   Black pepper
- Oats   Lima beans
- Peanuts   Pumpkin seeds
- Pork   Fish
- Sesame seeds   Turkey
- Brazil nuts   Mustard
- Paprika   Pecans
- Yeast   Lamb
- Soybeans   Wheat
- Almonds   Oysters
- Walnuts   Sardines

Herbs:

- Alfalfa   Cayenne   Dandelion   Skullcap
- Fennel Seed   Hops   Sage
- Wild Yam   Burdock Root

Symptoms of deficiency:

- Alopecia   Appetite Loss   Joint Problems   Fatigue
- Loss of taste Acne   Infertility

- Rashes   Diarrhea   Delayed wound healing

Facts:

- Zinc levels may be lowered by diarrhea, perspiration, diabetes and kidney disease

HERBS:

In 1820, the first edition of the United States Pharmacopeia was published. 67% of items in that book were herbal alternatives.

To create a herbal supplement, active ingredients are taken from the plant. Parts used include the berries, roots, stems, leaves, seeds, flowers and bark. Herbs are available for purchase in many forms; capsules, tablets, extracts, infusions, teas, decoctions, fresh plants, tinctures, glycerites, infused, essential oils and sprays.

∞ **Tincture:** Essences prepared by steeping in alcohol

∞ **Capsules:** Pill container that's filled with herbs or extract in a juice, powdered or oil form

∞ **Infusions/Teas:** Steeping in water

∞ **Glycerites:** Extracting herb with glycerite rather than water

∞ **Sprays:** Used for aromatherapy or topically

∞ **Extracts:** Retrieved by treating the herb with a solvent, such as alcohol

∞ **Decoctions:** Obtained by placing herb in boiling water

∞ **Ointments:** Herbs that are combined with a base, usually beeswax, Vaseline or oil

∞ **Essential Oils:** Extracted from the herb after the herb was distilled

∞ **Infused Oils:** Created by soaking the herb in oil that is warm over a certain amount of time

As previously mentioned in this chapter, all things labeled "natural" or "herbal" are not necessarily safe. With that in mind, how are you supposed to know what is good to take? There are a few ways to verify the safety of any product you are considering taking. The best way is to check a database. The National Center for Complementary and Alternative Medicine maintains lists on what each supplement is for, the side effects and how safe they are.

Here are some tips to help you use herbs safely:

✓ Don't take them if nursing or pregnant unless it has been indicated as safe

✓ Start small to test for any reactions, allergic or otherwise

✓ Use quality herbs from trust sellers/company/source

✓ Use for recommended period of time
✓ Ensure label contains recommended doses, directions, expiration date and lot number
✓ Review cautions and ingredients on label of container
✓ When in doubt, always consult a professional

The following is a list of herbs that are beneficial for use with PCOS symptoms. You'll find the herb name, the botanical name, what it is best used to treat and any additional important notes.

- ❖ Alfalfa   Botanical name: Medicago Sativa
  - o Lowers cholesterol   Stabilizes blood sugar and hormonal imbalances
  - o Anti-inflammatory   Diuretic

- ❖ Aloe   Botanical name: Aloe Vera
  - o Anti-fungal   Anti-bacterial   Anti-inflammatory   Lowers cholesterol

- ❖ Bergamont   Botanical name: Monarda Didyma
  - o Antiseptic   Antiemetic   Acne   Nausea   Insomnia
  - o Vomiting   Tension   Menstrual cramps

- ❖ Black Cohosh   Botanical name: CimiciFuga Racemosa
  - o Reduces PMS symptoms and menstrual cramps   Menopausal symptoms
  - o Reduces blood pressure and cholesterol   Depression

Black cohosh contains small amounts of salicyclic acid, therefor people who have aspirin allergies should not take Black Cohosh.

- ❖ Black Haw   Botanical name: Viburnum Prunifolium
  - o Reduces menstrual cramps   Helpful in preventing miscarriages

- ❖ Blessed Thistle   Botanical name: Cnicus Benedictus
  - o Stimulates appetite   Anti-inflammatory   Increases milk flow for nursing
  - o Cleanses the blood   Aids female disorders

- ❖ Blue Cohosh   Botanical name: Caulophyllum Thalictroides
  - o Eases painful menstruation, ovulation and childbirth   Amenorrhea

- ❖ Burdock   Botanical name: Arctium Lappa
  - o Antioxidant   Anti-bacterial   Anti-fungal   High in Vitamin C and Iron
  - o Acne   Toothache   Insomnia

- ❖ Calendula/Marigold   Botanical name: Calendula Officinalis
  - ○ Menstrual cramps   Regulates cycle   Acne
  - ○ Reduces swelling from cystic ovaries   Nausea
  - ○ Can possibly unblock fallopian tubes   Dry skin
  - ○ Anti-inflammatory   Stomach ache

- ❖ Chamomile   Botanical name: Matricaria Recutita
  - ○ Anti-inflammatory   Diuretic   Eases menstrual cramps   Stress   Anxiety

- ❖ Cinnamon Bark   Botanical name: Cinnamomum Verum
      PMS symptoms   Infertility   Restores appetite   Relieves diarrhea

- ❖ Cramp Bark   Botanical name: Viburnum Opulus
  - ○ Reduces pain from intestinal and menstrual cramps
  - ○ Reduces risk of miscarriage

- ❖ Dandelion   Botanical name: Taraxacum Officinale
  - ○ Lowers blood pressure   Relieves bloating and menstrual pain
  - ○ Anti-inflammatory   Antioxidant   Antibacterial
  - ○ Heartburn   Acne   Laxative   Lowers cholesterol
    The inside of the dandelion plan leaves is a mass amount of nutrients.
    Those include A, C, D, B complex, Iron, Zinc, Potassium and Calcium to
    name a few. Young leaves are also mixed into salad greens.

- ❖ Dong Quai   Botanical name: Angelica Sinensis
  - ○ Aids in strengthening blood in people with anemia   Sedative
  - ○ Laxative   Diuretic   Pain reliever   Vaginal dryness   hot flashes
  - ○ Helps with PMS symptoms, menopause, infertility, irregular menstruation
  - ○ Lowers blood pressure   Eases menstrual cramps

  Due to how often Dong Quai is used with gynecological problems, it is often
  called "female ginseng'. Headaches have been noted when used in high doses.
  Dong Quai should be avoided by people who are allergic to parsley, carrots or
  celery.

- ❖ Evening Primrose Oil   Botanical name: Oenothera Biennis
  - ○ Reduces PMS and breast tenderness   Lowers blood pressure

- o Eases hot flashes and menstrual cramps   Reduces heavy bleeding
- o Anti-inflammatory   Acne   Headache   Anxiety   Insomnia
- o Regulates menstrual cycles

- ❖ False Unicorn Root   Botanical name: Chamaelirium Luteum
  - o Eases menstrual cramps and menopause symptoms
  - o Helps female reproductive organ ailments (infertility, miscarriage)

- ❖ Fennel   Botanical name: Foeniculum Vulgare
  - o Nausea   Vomiting   Menstrual cramps   Anti-inflammatory

- ❖ Fenugreek   Botanical name: Trigonella Foenum Graecum)
  - o Lowers cholesterol   Laxative   Balances blood sugar
    Those who are allergic to chickpeas should not take fenugreek. Side
    effects noted are sweating and mild gastrointestinal upset.

- ❖ Feverfew   Botanical name: Tanacetum Parthenium
  - o Migraines   menstrual cramps   muscle tension
  - o Laxative   Depression   Insomnia   Regulates menstrual cycle
  - o Anti-inflammatory

If you suffer from an allergy to the following, you shouldn't take feverfew;
Ragweed, Yarrow, Marigold, Daisy or Chamomile. Handling the leaves may also
cause an allergic skin reaction.

- ❖ Garlic   Botanical name: Allium Sativum
  - o Lowers blood pressure and cholesterol
  - o Raises HDL levels   Boosts immune functions
  - o Menstrual cramps
  - o Antibacterial   Antifungal   Antioxidant

Side effects noted are heartburn, bloating, headache, nausea

- ❖ Gentian   Botanical name: Gentiana Lutea
  - o Regulates menstrual cycle   stimulates appetite   aids digestion
  - o Diarrhea   Nausea   Heartburn
  - o Anti-inflammatory

- ❖ Ginkgo   Botanical name: Ginkgo Biloba
  - o Anti-inflammatory   Antioxidant   Lowers cholesterol

- ❖ Hops   Botanical name: Humulus Lupulus
  - o Anxiety Insomnia Pain Toothaches Nervousness Stress
  - o Menstrual cramps Headache Irritability   Regulates menstrual cycle

- ❖ Jasmine   Botanical name: Jasminum Officinale
  - o Sedative   Headaches   Insomnia Tension Depression   Anxiety

- ❖ Juniper   Botanical name: juniperus communis
  - o Lowers blood pressure Regulates cycles Eases PMS symptoms   Diuretic

- ❖ Kava   Botanical name: Piper Methysticum
  - o Anxiety Insomnia Migraine Reduces pain and menstrual cramps

  Kava is metabolized by the liver which is why it is so toxic if used too much.

- ❖ Lady's Mantle   Botanical name: Alchemilla Vulgaris
  - o Anti-inflammatory   Diarrhea   Regulates menstrual cycle   Acne
  - o PMS   Menstrual cramps   Treats fibroids   Aids healthy conception
  - o Excessive menstrual bleeding   Helps body produce progesterone

- ❖ Lavender   Botanical name: Lavendula Angustifolia
  - o Headache Stress Anxiety Insomnia Depression Regulates cycle
  - o Sedative   Irritability

- ❖ Lemon Balm   Botanical name: Melissa Officinalis
  - o Anxiety Insomnia PMS symptoms Menstrual cramps Depression
  - o Headaches   Fatigue   Regulates menstrual cycle

- ❖ Maca   Botanical name: Lepidium Meyenii
  - o Fatigue Infertility Menopausal symptoms   Regulates menstrual cycle

- ❖ Marjoram   Botanical name: Origanum Vulgare
  - o Anti-inflammatory   Anxiety   Insomnia   Menstrual cramps
  - o Headache   Irritability

- ❖ Motherwort   Botanical name: Leonurus Cardiaca
  - o Helps with headaches, insomnia and vertigo   Reduces anxiety attacks
  - o Aids in female reproductive system Eases painful PMS and menstruation

. FUN FACT

The word Cardiaca comes from the Greek word meaning heart. It got the name because Motherwort has been used to correct heart palpitations as well as fast heartbeats (Tachycardia) since ancient times.

- ❖ Mugwort Leaf   Botanical name: Artemesia Vulgaris
  - o Menstrual cramps   Depression   Reduces excessive menstrual bleeding
  - o Regulates cycle   Anti-inflammatory   Sedative

- ❖ Passion Flower   Botanical name: Passiflora Incarnata
  - o Stress Insomnia Anxiety PMS symptoms Lowers blood pressure
  - o Tension   Hysteria   Headache   Irritability

- ❖ Raspberry   Botanical name: Rubus Idaeus
  - o Diarrhea   Menstrual cramps   Fatigue   Depression
  - o Hot flashes   Excessive menstrual bleeding
  - o Regulate menstrual cycle   Antioxidant   PMS
  - o High in calcium, potassium and Vitamin C

- ❖ Rose   Botanical name: Rosa spp.
  - o Headache   Raise sperm count   Regulate hormones   Depression
  - o Menstrual cramps   Regulate menstrual cycle   Infertility
  - o High in Vitamin C

- ❖ Rosemary   Botanical name: Rosmarinus Officinalis
  - o Headaches Depression Fatigue Menstrual cramps Antioxidant
  - o Weak circulation   Restores appetite   Regulates menstrual cycle
  - o Reduces risk of cancer and heart disease   Promotes hair growth

- ❖ Rhubarb   Botanical name: Rheum Officinale
  - o Regulates menstrual cycles   Headaches   Diarrhea

- ❖ Saw Palmetto   Botanical name: Serenoa Repens
  - o Reduces acne   Eases endocrine related disorders   raises sperm count
  - o Appetite stimulant

- ❖ Shepherd's purse   Botanical name: Capsella Bursa-Pastoris
  - o Reduces/ stops profuse menstrual bleeding

  Young leaves can be eaten in salad greens

- ❖ Skullcap   Botanical name: Scutellaria Lateriflora
    - o Stress   Anxiety   Tension   Depression   Hysteria   Insomnia
    - o Headache   Menstrual cramps

- ❖ Soy Isoflavone   Botanical name: Gylcine max
    - o Lowers cholesterol   Eases menopausal and PMS symptoms

- ❖ St. John's Wort   Botanical name: Hypericum Perforatum
    - o Anxiety   Depression   Insomnia   Diarrhea   Menstrual cramps
      St. John's Wort may interfere with anti-depressants and oral contraceptives.

- ❖ Tea Tree   Botanical name: Melaleuca Alternifolia
    - o Eases acne, boils, cuts and wounds   Relieves sore throat and mouth sores

- ❖ Turmeric   Botanical name: Curcuma Longa
    - o Eases menstrual pain   Regulates menstrual cycle
    - o Antibiotic and anti-inflammatory

- ❖ Valerian   Botanical name: Valeriana Officinalis
    - o Insomnia   Anxiety   Reduces headaches and menstrual cramps   Stress
    - o Sedative   Lower blood pressure   Acne
      Valerian can possibly interact with anesthesia therefor it should be stopped at least 24 hours before surgery.

FUN FACT
<u>Considered the Valium of the nineteenth century</u>

- ❖ Vervain (Verbena Officinalis)
    - o Depression   Regulates menstrual cycle   Eases menstrual cramps
    - o Eases headache   Stress   Insomnia   Tension

- ❖ Vitex   Botanical name: vitex agnus-castus /Chasteberry
    - o Restores menstruation and ovulation   Corrects hormonal imbalances
    - o Eases PMS symptoms and hot flashes   Reduces acne

Side effects noted are headaches, upset stomach, and fatigue. Vitex should not be taken with any hormones (estrogen or progesterone), medications that alter endocrine activity or that interfere with prolactin levels.

FUN FACT

Ancient Greeks & Romans believed Vitex promoted chastity and it was used to suppress sexual desire which is where it received its name chasteberry from.

- ❖ White Willow   Botanical name: Salix Alba AKA: Willow Bark.
    - o   Headaches   Menstrual cramps   Anti-inflammatory

- ❖ Wild Oats   Botanical name: Avena Fatua
    - o   Eases lower abdominal pain   helps with depression

- ❖ Wild Yam   Botanical name: Dioscorea Villosa
    - o   Eases nausea and morning sickness   Eases PMS symptoms
    - o   Reduces menstrual cramps, intestinal and uterine spasms

- ❖ White Willow   Botanical name: Salix Alba AKA: Willow Bark.
    - o   Headaches   Menstrual cramps   Anti-inflammatory

- ❖ Wormwood   Botanical name: Artemesia Absinthium
    - o   Anti-inflammatory   Anxiety   Depression   Stimulates uterus

- ❖ Yarrow   Botanical name: Achillea Millefolium
    - o   Reduces menstruation pain   Lowers fever   Lowers blood pressure
    - o   Acne   Diarrhea   Regulates menstrual cycle   UTI
    - o   Irritability   Anti-inflammatory

FUN FACT

was said to be the favorite herb of Achilles. He used Yarrow during the Trojan War as a treatment for wounds.

Herb Terms:

- Abortifacient: Causes miscarriage Ex: Pennyroyal
- Adaptogen: Helps body adapt to stress Ex: Ginseng
- Alterative: Helps improve general health by balancing body functions Ex: Burdock
- Anticatarrhal: Lowers mucous production Ex: Goldenseal
- Antidepressant: Relieves depression feelings Ex: St. John's Wort
- Antidote: Counteracts effects of poison
- Anti-emetic: Prevents vomiting Ex: Ginger
- Antifungal: Eliminates fungus
- Antigalactic: Reduces breast milk secretions Ex: Sage
- Antihelmintic: Destroys parasites Ex: Garlic
- Anti-inflammatory: Reduces inflammation Ex: Black Cohosh
- Antioxidant: Prevents damage of cells by free radicals Ex: Milk Thistle
- Antipyretic: Reduces fever Ex: Yarrow
- Antispasmodic: Reduces muscle spasms Ex: Kava
- Carminative: Reduces gas Ex: Fennel
- Cathartic: Laxative Ex: Rhubarb
- Diaphoretic: Causes perspiration Ex: Yarrow
- Diuretic: Promotes urination Ex: Dandelion
- Emetic: Causes vomiting Ex: Ipecac
- Febrifuge: Lowers fever Ex: White Willow
- Galactagogue: Promotes milk flow Ex: Fennel
- Hemostatic: Stops bleeding Ex: Yarrow
- Hypnotic: Induces sleep Ex: Valerian
- Hypotensive: Lowers blood pressure Ex: Garlic
- Sedative: Calming Ex: Valerian

CHAPTER 9 -COMPLEMENTARY MEDICINE

These are methods that are used while using traditional medicine. Complementary medicine is basically an umbrella phrase; it encompasses many techniques that offer healing. Treatments focus on healing the body as a whole and finding the root cause rather than just treating the symptoms. We will touch on a few, but there are many different forms of complementary medicine available to you.

- Acupressure   Acupuncture   Aromatherapy   Ayurveda
- Bodywork   Chiropractic   Flower Essences   Homeopathy
- Hydrotherapy   Hypnotherapy   Naturopathy   Supplements
- Qigong   Reflexology   Reiki   Relaxation/Meditation
- Tai Chi   Massage   Trigger Point Therapy   Yoga

Acupressure:

Acupressure works off of the belief that our body has certain pathways called "meridians" that run throughout it. An energy called "Qi" (pronounced Chee) flows in the meridians. However certain things like stress, unhealthy eating and no exercise are a few things that can cause congestion in our meridians and mess up the flow of our Qi.

Acupressure sessions involve finger pressure, much like a massage, in areas where our Qi is blocked from flowing freely. It is a way to allow our body to be able to heal itself.

Acupressure been found to help your body release chemicals called endorphins. These help to reduce pain, panic and anxiety as well as help muscles to relax.

Helps to treat:

- Anxiety Migraines Stress Depression Hormonal Imbalances
- Dizziness PMS Symptoms Insomnia And more

Acupuncture:

Acupuncture holds the same beliefs as acupressure. Very similar expect acupuncture involves inserting tiny needles into your skin in select areas instead of massaging them with your hands. In 1996 these needles were officially classified as a medical device by the FDA which in turn enabled more insurance companies to begin paying for acupuncture treatments.

The needles that are used today vary in length, typically ½ inch to 3 inches.

FUN FACT
<u>Many years ago the needles used for acupuncture were made from slivers of bone or bamboo that had been sharpened.</u>

Acupuncture is beneficial in treating more problems than acupressure, including:

- o Acne   Diabetes   High Blood Pressure   Impotence
- o Infertility   Menstrual Irregularities   Anxiety   Diarrhea
- o Hormonal Imbalances   Hypoglycemia   Depression
- o Menstrual cramps   Headaches   Insomnia   Stress
- o And more

Acupuncturists should have completed a minimum of a three year course; however exact requirements for licensing vary in every state.

For more information and a list of referrals for practitioners that are licensed or registered nationwide, contact American Association of Acupuncture and Oriental Medicine

Naturopathy:

Naturopathy is about the body having the ability to heal itself. You're viewed as a whole instead of one particular symptom. Naturopaths specialize in natural medicine and have training in various areas including acupuncture, nutrition, counseling, homeopathy, hydrotherapy, and more. This enables them to treat any condition or symptom that you would see your primary doctor about.

John Scheel first invented the term naturopathy in 1895. He was a physician from New York City who ended up selling the term "Naturopathy" to Benedict Lust. In 1902 Benedict Lust, an immigrant from Germany founded a naturopathy school in New York City. He called it The American School of Naturopathy.

Helps to treat:

- o High Cholesterol   Depression   Headache   High Blood Pressure
- o Insomnia   Menstrual problems   Nausea   Pain   Stress and more

Chiropractic:

Chiropractors believe that an aligned spine is how to continue optimal health. They manipulate your spine which allows for proper functioning of the nervous system. This enables the signals to go out like they are supposed to do. Think of it like this; you pull up to the drive through window at the bank and the teller sends the container down the pipe. In this instance the bank teller is your brain, the pipe is your spine and the container is your spinal cord which delivers messages to your body. If your spine is not aligned the right way, you can't get the messages. Most insurance plans have some sort of chiropractic coverage.

Chiropractors are able to treat many conditions such as:

- Ankle Swelling   Diarrhea   Fatigue   Insomnia   Allergies
- Back Pain   Constipation   Headaches   Low Blood Pressure
- High Blood Pressure Dizziness   Menstrual Problems   PMS
- And more

Chiropractic care began in 1895. It was then that a man by the name of Daniel David Palmer from Davenport, Iowa healed a deaf man and restored his hearing. The deaf man, a janitor, had lost his hearing many years prior when heard a loud pop from his back. Daniel Palmer had noticed one of his vertebras was not in the correct position. Once pushed back to the intended place, his hearing came back.

Chiropractor comes from the Greek words Cheir which means hand and Praxis which means practice / Practikos which means done by.

"If you would seek health, look first to the spine."
-- Socrates

Therapeutic touch:

Back in 1970, Dolores Krieger RN, Ph.D. and Dora Kunz, a healer, developed therapeutic touch.

They believe every person has a field of energy around them. It covers their entire body and protrudes out many inches above our skin.

Aside from what the name implies, therapeutic touch doesn't involve touching our bodies. They touch our energy field as a way of healing our energy to enable the body to heal itself.

Therapeutic touch helps:

- Pain   Anxiety   Relaxation   Nervous Disorder
- High Blood Pressure   Menstrual Problems   And more

Homeopathy:

In the 1790's, a German physician by the name of Samuel Hahnermann, developed homeopathy. It is based upon the principle that a substance that can create particular symptoms in a person can cure the same symptoms.

This is where homeopathy got its name from. Homeo is a Greek word that means "like" and pathos means "suffering."

Homeopathy helps:

- Anxiety   Digestive Problems   Pain   Headaches   Insomnia
- Endocrine Disorders   Menstrual Problems   PMS   and more

Beneficial Homeopathic remedies:

- Chamomilla- Painful periods, cramping, irritability
- Ipecac- Nausea, vomiting, menstrual problems
- Sepia- Hair loss, headaches, hot flashes, menstrual cramps
- Aconitum Napellus- Fear, anxiety
- Aloe Socotrina- Digestive problems
- Argentum Nitricum- Anxiety
- Aurum Metallicum- Depression
- Bryonia Alba- Headaches
- Cantharis Vesicatoria- Urinary tract infections
- Caulo Phyllum- Female organ issues
- Cimacifuga- Delayed menstruation
- Cuprum Metallicum- Cramps
- Kali Carbonicum- Headaches
- Kreosotum- Anxiety, female organ issues

- Mangesia Muriatica- Depression, anxiety, cramps
- Magnesia Phosphorica- Cramps, headaches
- Viburnum Opulus- Cramps

Relaxation:

This goes hand in hand with meditation. It offers relief from the same ailments however, relaxation has different techniques.

- Autogenic Training- Encompasses the same idea of the childhood game "light as a feather, stiff as a board." Basically you trick your mind. You would repeat phrases about your body, listing each part differently to achieve your ultimate goal of relaxation. For example, "my right arm is warm."
- Progressive Muscle Relaxation- involves tensing and relaxing each part of your body. Close your eyes and inhale. Start with the muscles toward the top of your body. One at a time, clench and hold for 5-10 seconds. Release and exhale. This technique can help with insomnia, pms, high blood pressure and infertility to name a few.

Reiki:

Pronounced Ray-Key, it is the art of light touch massage. It comes from the Japanese words Rei and Ki. Rei means "universal spirit" while Ki means "life force energy."

Reiki is about restoring your body's flow of its healing energies. It involves physical, emotional, psychological and spiritual healing. It is a Tibetan Buddhist practice that has been around for well over 2,000 years. A few conditions that reiki is helpful with are:

- Anxiety Emotional problems Fatigue Reproductive Disorders
- Stress related disorders

They believe we have energy surrounding our body called chakras. The Reiki Master places their hands over these chakras and channels energy into it thus ridding your body of its old energy. This is supposed to heal your body's cells and enable proper functioning of its systems.

Kyo Dake Wa (Kee Oh dah Kay Wah) means Just Today

Shinpai Suna (Shin-pie soo nah) means Don't Worry

These are 2 of the 5 Reiki Spiritual Priniciples

Reflexology:

Reflexology is a special massage for feet, hands and ears, developed in the mid 1930's by Eunice Ingham a physical therapist from Rochester, NY. It reduces stress and stress related health problems. It is believed that our hands and feet are the mirrors of our body.

Certain areas on each hand and foot are linked to other body parts. For instance:

The right foot helps the right side of the body

The left foot helps the left side of the body

The big toe helps the head and brain

The soles of your feet help your organs and glands

The ankle and heel of your foot help your pelvic area, bladder and reproductive organs

A reflexology treatment is fairly simple. The reflexologist will apply pressure and stimulation to the reflex areas that correspond to specific organ systems to locate and correct the problems in your body. The goal is to restore the natural flow of energy in the zones on our body. Our bodies are divided into 10 equal zones.

Reflexology helps to treat:

- Allergies Cramps Constipation Fatigue Headaches Insomnia
- High Blood Pressure Lack of energy Nausea PMS symptoms
- Stress related disorders Blocked or damaged fallopian tubes

Reflexology has been found helpful in regulating hormones to improve menstrual cycles, help with menopause and even aid in conception.

Massage:

Massage is the manual manipulation by a masseuse of the soft tissue and muscles to help relax.

Massage comes from the French word Masser which means "to knead" and the Sanskrit word Makeh which means "to press softly."

In the Egyptian tomb of Ankhmahr built around 2200 BC and known as the tomb of the physician, one of the wall paintings depicts two men having their extremities treated with massage.

Massage can be helpful in treating many ailments such as:

- Improving immunity   Improving circulation   Stress   Headaches
- Migraines   Back pain   Sore muscles   PMS   Depression   Insomnia

Ayurveda:

This is a system that is over 5,000 years old, which loosely translates to the science of life. Ayurvedic medicine believes each person has a dominant energy in them and through that dominant energy they can be healed. This energy is called a "dosha" which means body type. Ayurvedic Medicine comes from Veda meaning knowledge and Ayus meaning life.

There are three dosha types.

- ✧ Vata – air and space
- ✧ Pitta – fire and water
- ✧ Kapha – water and earth

Below are lists of characteristics of each dosha. The one you relate to the most is your dominant dosha.

- ✧ Vata: dry curly hair. Thin bony physique. Dry skin. Vivacious, imaginative. Dislikes cold. Light sleeper. Intuitive. Easily fatigued. Quick to learn and forget. Anxious under stress.
- ✧ Pitta: thin, fine hair. Medium muscled build. Ruddy, freckled complexion. Fiery and intense. Dislikes the heat. Moderate sound sleeper. Strong and articulate. Medium mental capacity. Irritated under stress.

✧ Kapha: dark full hair. Heavy set, curvy. Strong. Oily, smooth skin. Steady, slow. Dislikes damp and cold. Heavy sleeper. Compassionate. High stamina. Slow to learn, good memory. Relaxed under stress.

Ayurveda helps to treat many disorders:

- Dermatological   Emotional   Endocrine   Immune   Nervous
- Reproductive   Cardiovascular

Hypnotherapy:

Hypnosis is the induction of a deeply relaxed trance like state, followed by used of suggestion. The word hypnosis is from a Greek word hypnos which means "to sleep."

FUN FACT

Did you know the word mesmerize comes from a doctor? Dr. Franz Anton Mesmer. He is considered a founder of hypnotherapy.

You cannot be forced into a hypnotic state against your will. The motivation to participate in treatment and hope that treatment will be effective are essential factors in benefiting from hypnosis.

Hypnosis can help:

- Addictions   Anxiety   Behavioral Problems   Endocrine Disorders
- Fears   Hypertension   Insomnia   Phobias   Migraines
- Weight Problems   Stress related problems

Guided Imagery and Visualization:

This is the art of promoting relaxation by visualizing it. It is essential to have an open mind when you are attempting to reach goals and fix conditions.

Think about your ovaries, covered in cysts. Envision them enlarged and frustratingly disobedient.

Imagery is about using your senses; sight, sound, smell and touch.

Keep your envisioned ovaries in mind. Now watch a hand come in with a giant pin. It begins to pop each and every one. Hear them pop like a balloon. See the fluid burst out when they explode. See your body healed, with no remaining cysts.

The object is to use these images in a positive way that will encourage certain actions to take place within the body. Guided imagery may not be enough to cure a condition; however it may put you in a better state of mind which enable you to cope better. Just as an asthmatic won't be cured, guided imagery will give them the ability to calm their breathing to control the symptoms.

Meditation:

When you head that word, do you think of sitting criss cross on the floor, dim room and relaxing music playing? I do. It doesn't have to be exactly like that though. It's really about finding an inner peace, wherever and however you do it best. There are different kinds of meditation. Let's touch briefly on a few.

- ✧ Vibrational: (also called sounding meditation) this has a word or sound as its main focal point through repetition called a mantra.
- ✧ Journey: this enables you to find peace by using imagery and visualization to put yourself "in peace."
- ✧ Mindfulness: This encourages you to focus on what's going on around you at that point in time. This allows you to take the time to enjoy life without judgement.

No matter which way you prefer, meditation can treat many disorders such as:

- o Cardiovascular Dermatological Nervous Digestive Respiratory
- o Reproductive Immune Anxiety Headaches Asthma Pain
- o Stress High Blood Pressure

it can help so many conditions due to the reduction of stress. High levels of stress can worsen the symptoms of many things.

Hydrotherapy:

German farmer Vincent Preissnitz started using wet compresses in the early 1800's. He used them to heal his broken ribs after he was ran over by a wagon when he was 17 years old. He discovered water could help the body heal. Hydrotherapy is any form of water based treatment. It works excellently on conditions where circulation is impaired also that cause muscle weakness. Menstrual cramps, PMS, stress, inflammation and diabetes are great candidates.

Aquatic therapy involves water as well except this is exercising and stretching in the water.

Ways we use hydrotherapy today:

- o Hot packs   Cold packs   Sitz baths   Whirlpool   Hot tub
- o Saunas   Ice massage   Jacuzzi

Flower Essences:

Using flower essences to heal was a practice discovered in England during the 1930's by Edward Bach, a homeopath physician.

The belief is that if our mental or emotional state is imbalanced, or physical state will be unable to defend and heal itself. For this reason, when picking which essence to use, you are asked to not think about physical illness and instead focus on how you are feeling mentally.

Bach thought flowers had healing or soothing properties in them, which led to making remedies from the flowers essence. He has 38 remedies plus a rescue remedy. You can purchase the remedies over the counter and used them daily without addiction concerns or bad side effects. They can be ingested directly under your tongue or even in a drink of choice because they are incredibly diluted solutions. If you'd rather, you can apply it to the temples or other body parts.

Using flower essences helps to treat:

- o Anxiety   Stress   Internal Conflicts   Grief   Depression   PMS
- o Headache   Insomnia   and more

Flower essence treatments are not there for preventing emotional problems, just to help relieve the existing ones.

Flower essences contain no parts of the flower; they are only the liquid extracts. The 38 Bach flower essences are:

- Agrimony: mental torture, to hide feelings
- Aspen: Eases anxiety of unknown
- Beech: Intolerance, become more accepting
- Centaury: Helps you to say no, for the easily influenced
- Cerato: Believe in your decisions, for over dependency
- Cherry plum: Helps you to stay in control
- Chestnut Bud: Failure to learn from mistakes, help breaking habits
- Chicory: Helps with possessiveness and being controlling
- Clematis: Daydreaming, helps to ground you
- Crab apple: Improves self-worth
- Elm: Overwhelmed by responsibility, helps you "feel ready"
- Pine: Guilt
- Gentian: Discouragement after a setback, become resilient
- Gorse: Hopelessness, helps you to keep going
- Heather: self-centeredness
- Holly: Hatred, envy, jealousy, heals hurt feelings
- Hornbeam: Procrastination
- Honeysuckle: Living in the past
- Impatiens: Impatience
- Larch: Lack of confidence
- Mimulus: Comforts anxiety
- Mustard: Deep gloom for no reason
- Oak: Exhaustion
- Olive: Exhaustion following effort, improves energy
- Red Chestnut: Overly concerned with loved ones welfare
- Rockrose: Terror
- Scleranthus: Inability to choose
- Star of Bethleham: Shock, grief
- Sweet Chestnut: Extreme mental anguish, improves hope
- Vervain: Over enthusiasm
- Vine: Dominance and inflexibility
- Walnut: Protection from unwanted influences
- Water Violet: Pride and aloofness
- White Chestnut: Unwanted thoughts and mental arguments
- Wild Oat: Uncertainty over lifes direction
- Wild Rose: drifting, apathy

- Willow: Self-pity, resentment
- Rescue Remedy: Star of Bethlehem, Rock Rose, Impatiens, Cherry Plum, Clematis = Helps with terror and stress

Aroma Therapy:

Using essentials oils to help relieve stress from physical, mental and emotional problems is known as aroma therapy. These oils have been extracted from certain plants using the leaves, seeds, flowers, grass, wood, fruit, roots, resins and herbs. Each oil has distinct healing energy. The oils can either be applied directly to you skin or inhaled. However due to the high level of concentration, they should not be taken internally as it can lead to a toxic overdose.

Aroma therapy oils can be made into an ointment, compress and bath oils. They can also be used during massages or in a vaporizer system.

While the exact amounts used vary, the following doses are pretty common.

1-2 drops to smell or in perfume

2-3 drops on a rag in a drawer

2 drops per ½ cup of water for a compress

3-4 drops in a pot of hot water to inhale

4-5 drops in a bath

3-5 drops in 1 oz of skin cream

15 drops per 1oz of oil for massage oil

FUN FACT

Did you know in 1928 French chemist Rene-Mauric Gattefosse coined the term "aromatherapie"

Aromatherapy helps treat:

- Anxiety Fatigue Insomnia Constipation Headaches
- Nausea Depression Hormonal imbalance PMS symptoms

- And more

Aromatherapy is effective because smell is directly connected to your brain. Your brain controls the ANS which is why you react to smell without even thinking about it.

If you apply the essential oil of your choice to the bottom of your foot it will work faster because of how fast the oils get absorbed and make their way into your blood stream. You can also apply the oils to your temples, behind your ears and your ear lobes. You can also dilute the essential oil by adding another type of oil or water to it. The best oils to add are almond, apricot, grapeseed, jojoba, or olive oil.

Carrier Oils:

- Almond Oil: Relieves inflammation
- Apricot kernel Oil: Best for dry skin. Full of Vitamin A
- Avocado Oil: Best for problems with skin. Full of Vitamin A & E
- Canola Oil: Stores very well
- Evening Primrose Oil: Best for skin repair
- Flaxseed Oil: Full of Vitamin E
- Grapeseed Oil: Great for acne ridden skin
- Hazelnut Oil: Promotes firmness of skin
- Jojoba Oil: Hydrates skin
- Olive Oil: Blends well
- Sunflower Oil: Best for sensitive skin

If you ever have any questions, you should contact a qualified aroma therapist.

There are also many helpful books out there such as:

Aroma Therapy 101 by Karen Downes

Aromatherapy an illustrated guide by Clare Walters

Aroma Therapy oils beneficial for PCOS:

- Bergamont (citrus bergamia) Used as an anti-depressant, balancing, calming, sedative, acne, anxiety and insomnia. Bergamont has anti- septic properties making it good for skin and scalp conditions.

FUN FACT

<u>Named after the town in Italy where it was cultivated, Bergamo</u>

- Atlas Cedarwood (Cedrus Altantica) Used as an anti-depressant, strengthening, meditation, acne, alopecia, grounding, anxiety, dandruff and dry skin

FUN FACT
Word cedar originated from the Arabic Kedron. It means power.

- Cypress (Cupressus Sempervirens) Used for anxiety, comforting, regulates heavy and or painful menstruation; antifungal relieves sorrow, balances female reproductive system, and counteracts fatigue.

FUN FACT
Sempervirens means "lives forever"

- Clary sage (Salvia Sclarea) Used as a sedative, irritability, balancing the female reproductive system and endocrine system, eases menstrual pain and PMS symptoms, anxiety, stress, depression and relieves sorrow. Clary sage is referred to as feminine oil. Has an antioxidant and anti-inflammatory property.

FUN FACT
Dates back to ancient Egypt to cure infertility

- Roman Chamomile (Chamaemelum Nobile) used for insomnia, PMS symptoms, comforting stress, anxiety, inflammation, healing, soothing, tension, regulates menstrual cycles, reduces menstrual cramps
- Geranium (Pelargonium Graveolens) Used to balance hormones, helps with heavy menstruation, pms symptoms and depression
- Ylang- ylang (Cananga Odorata) used to lower blood pressure, balance hormones and reproductive system, helps with depression, stress, insomnia, anxiety, alopecia, and acne.
- Sweet marjoam (Origanum Majorana) used for anxiety, stress, comforting, insomnia, migraines, menstrual pain, relieve sorrow and regulates cycle
- Lavender (Lavandula Augustifolia) used for acne, alopecia, anxiety, depression, stress, insomnia, calming, painful menstruation, restores balance to systems, improves memory
- Jasmine (Jasminum Officinale) used as an anti-depressant, balance hormones, eases menstrual pain, increase spermatozoa and improve memory. Jasmine has antioxidant and antibacterial properties.
- Neroli (Citrus Aurantium) Used for stress, depression, insomnia, acne, stress marks, headaches, pms symptoms

FUN FACT
Named after Princess Anne Marie from Nerula, Italy. It was her favorite scent to wear.

- Sandalwood (Santalum Album) used for anxiety, stress, depression, insomnia, reproductive system, acne, aphrodisiac

- Rose (Rosa Centifolia) Used for depression, grief, anxiety, aphrodisiac, nausea, vomiting, regulates menstrual cycle, pms symptoms, stress, insomnia
- Tangerine (Citrus Reticulata) used for acne, depression, insomnia, pms symptoms, fluid retention
- Myrrh (Commiphora Myrrha) used for anxiety, antiseptic, anti-inflammatory, stress, insomnia
- Melissa / lemon balm (Melissa Officinalis) used for depression, stress, insomnia, regulates cycle, menstrual pain, grief, migraines, lowers blood pressure, alopecia, anxiety, balances emotions
- Frankincense (Boswellia Carteri) used for stress, anti-inflammatory, insomnia, reduces heavy menstruation, depression
- Grapefruit (citrus paradisi) used for acne, antioxidant, alopecia, stress , depression, headaches, pms symptoms
- Vetiver (Vetiveria Zizanoides) used as a tonic to the reproductive system, for acne, anxiety, depression, insomnia
- Yarrow (Achillea Millefolium) used to balance menstrual cycle flow, decreases cramps, alopecia, insomnia, blood pressure, anti-inflammatory, diuretic.
- Tarragon used for pms symptoms

Oils for Anxiety relief:

- Hyssop Orange Peach Spiced Apple Violet Leaf

Oils for Depression:

- Lemon Lemon Verbena Orange Petitgrain

Oils to improve memory:

- Rosemary Lemon

Oils to relieve sorrow:

- Fir Sage Rosemary

Oils for stress and insomnia:

- Chamomile Cinnamon Cloves Hops Nutmeg Orange
- Valerian Vanilla Violet

Oils to wake you up:

- Angelica Benzoin Black Pepper Fennel Lemon Peppermint o   Pine   Sage   Spiced Apple

-Oils of Arnica, basil, Clary Sage, Cypress, Juniper, Myrrh, Sage and Thyme should be avoided during pregnancy as they can possibly cause the uterus to contract.

Oils for Oily Skin: Juniper, Patchouli, Peppermint, Tea Tree, Ylang Ylang

Oils for Dry Skin: Fennel, Cedarwood, Rose, Jasmine, Neroli, Lavender

Oils for Dry Hair: Chamomile, Lavender, Rosemary

Oils for Dandruff: Tea Tree, Cedarwood, Rosemary, Pine

Aroma Therapy Conversion Chart

drops	tsp	Oz	Dram	Milliliter
8	1/10	1/6	1/3	½
10	1/8	1/48	1/6	5/8
20	¼	1/24	1/3	1 ¼
40	½	1/12	2/3	2 ½
TSP	TBSP	OZ	DRAM	ML
1	1/3	1/6	1 1/3	5
1 ½	½	¼	2	7 ½
3	1	½	4	15
6	2	1	8	30
24	8	4	½ Cup	120
48	16	8	1 cup / ½ pint	240
96	32	16	2cup/ 1 pint	480

CHAPTER 10- FERTILITY TREATMENT OPTIONS

ART stands for Assisted Reproductive Technology. There are many options to choose from; IVF, GIFT, ZIFT, surrogacy, egg donation, embryo donation, etc. Out of them all, IVF is the most common type of procedure.

ART procedures typically involve removing eggs, fertilizing them and transferring them back into the body. Each treatment comes with its own price tag. Before deciding on which kind is best for you, ask the office for the advantages, disadvantages and price sheet.

When you decide to undergo fertility treatments, you need to establish a plan. Decisions can always change but you should have a general idea about what treatments you will and will not do, also how long you're willing to try them. Emotional preparation is a big part of it as well. Every day we go to sleep praying to see our BFP tomorrow all the while not being sure if it will ever come. Once you are ready to begin and you have a doctor you're comfortable with, take a look at your finances. Nothing about fertility treatments are cheap unfortunately; however there are plenty of resources available to you. It is wise to do plenty of research and stay informed about your options.

At the end of the day, you are the one who is 100% responsible for your body and your health. Your physicians do what they think is best but no one knows your body like you know your body.

When you are looking for a center to provide any type of fertility treatment, here are some questions to ask:

- How long has the facility been open?
- Is there a waiting list? If so, how long?
- What does a procedure cost?
- What is included in that fee?
- Can I get a breakdown of costs involved?
- How many women has your facility treated?
- When and how are payments due?
- Do you have sperm and or eggs from donors there?
- Administrative fees to start cycle?
- Fees for all physicians you'll see?
- Fees for initial testing (hiv, hep test, cmv test, bacterial culture, etc)?

- What happens to left over embryos?
    - What are your success rates?
- What happens if the first cycle doesn't work?
    - Fees for initial evaluation (semen analysis, etc)?
    - Fees for ovulation induction (drugs and monitoring)?
- Fees for blood testing and ultrasounds as well as how many times each will happen per cycle?
    - Fees for HCG stimulation?
    - Fees to collect eggs?
    - Fees to freeze embryo?
    - Fees to store embryo?
    - Fees to transfer embryo?

Having the answers to even some of these questions will give you a huge advantage to planning which type of procedure you would like to have. There are many options available to you. While some are fairly similar, they do have a few differences among them.

Believe it or not, there is a science to sperm!

Approximately 10 million sperm make it to the vagina.

100,000 or less make it to the cervix

2,000 or less go to the CORRECT fallopian tube

200 or less get to the distal fallopian tube

10 or less make it to the egg

ONE achieves fertilization

Once sperm is inside your reproductive tract, it can survive for up to SEVEN days.

There are many options available to you. Let's take a look at a few.

- ✧ ZIFT (Zygote Intrafallopian Transfer) A ZIFT is also referred to as a TET (Tubal Embryo Transfer). Similar to an IVF treatment. After fertilization has occurred, the zygote (fertilized embryo) is then placed into your fallopian tube. It differs from IVF because during a IVF treatment the embryo is transferred into your uterus. Unfortunately in order for a ZIFT to be successful, fallopian tubes must be healthy and unblocked. To begin the process, ovaries are stimulated with medication to produce eggs. The eggs are collected, fertilized and then transferred with a laparoscopic procedure within 24 hours. While the cost will vary depending upon many factors, average price tag is $15,000- $20,000 per attempt.

- ✧ GIFT (Gamete Intrafallopian Transfer) a GIFT procedure is done via an all-natural cycle meaning they give you no drugs to stimulate ovulation. Once your eggs are mature, the physician removes them from your ovaries. Those eggs and sperm from your partner or a donor are then placed into your fallopian tube where your egg has the best chance of getting fertilized. Average price per GIFT attempt is $15,000- $20,000.

- ✧ IVM (InVitro Maturation) Egg follicles that are close to being mature are removed prior to ovulation. No medication is given to induce ovulation. Said follicles are left to finish maturing in a lab. Two are then implanted. This does not come with the side effects or high risk of OHSS like IVF does. IVM is beneficial for women who are susceptible to developing OHSS or in couples where the infertility is only a male factor.

- ✧ IUI (Intrauterine Insemination) IUI is a process that separates fast moving sperm from slow moving sperm. Given fertility medications to induce ovulation. Sperm is then injected directly into your uterus close to the time of ovulation which is usually 24-36 hours after the LH surge. This treatment option is often the first choice for many couples because it is much cheaper than other ART alternatives. The price will vary on many factors such as what facility you use, if you use donor sperm, your location throughout the world. The average cost is around $1500- $4000 per cycle. This usually includes ultrasound monitoring and medication.

- ✧ IVF (In Vitro Fertilization) , Average cost is $10,000- $20,000 per cycle. A cycle of IVF includes removing your eggs, transferring them to a petri dish. They are then incubated with sperm between 1-2 days. After they become fertilized, they are watched for a couple days (usually 3-5 days) or so to insure they have developed normally. If they have, then a few are transferred into your uterus. IVF was originally referred to as having "test tube babies." First IVF baby born in Oldham, England was in 1978 because of Dr. Patrick Steptoe. The first IVF baby born in Australia was in 1980. The first IVF baby born in USA was in 1981. (1)

There are risks associated with inducing ovulation. The biggest one is Ovarian Hyperstimulation Syndrome (OHSS). OHSS happens when ovaries respond too well to the induction medication. A few things can increase your chances of getting OHSS. They are: if you have PCOS, high estradiol levels, you're under 25 years of age, you're below normal weight, you've had OHSS previously or if you are using a high dose of drugs trying to induce ovulation. The signs to keep an eye out for are:

- Pain and or discomfort in your lower abdominal or pelvic area
- Bloating
- Weight Gain

Deciding to use a surrogate can mean a few things. You can choose to use her eggs, your eggs or even donor eggs from someone else. The same goes for sperm. Will you use your significant others sperm or a donor sperm? Those are some things to think about before moving forward with the process of using a surrogate.

- Gestational Surrogacy: Estimated cost of $30,000-$50,000 per cycle
- Traditional Surrogacy: Estimated cost of $22,500-$33,500 per cycle.

- Sperm Donation: When using sperm from an anonymous donor, the sperm should be frozen for a minimum of 180 days before you use it. This time frame will allow ample time to have the donor retested for infections he might have had when he donated that went undiagnosed like HIV
- Embryo Donation: Embryos are fertilized eggs that need a womb to implant and grow
- Egg Donation: If egg donation is the way you have decided to go, you'll need to think about where you want to get your eggs from. Some people use family members (Aunts, cousins, sisters, etc) while others pick a friend or close acquaintance. Both of these options are nice because not only will you get to know the source of your eggs, they also usually do not expect payment in return

so you may only need to cover medical costs. In the event you have no egg donor from above sources, you can always get one through a program that recruits donors. The estimated cost is $6,000-$20,000. Egg donation has been around since 1983. There are so many good reasons to consider using donor eggs, in the end the choice is yours. If you suffer from multiple miscarriages, absence of ovaries, have a poor response to fertility drugs, are going through menopause or even have a hereditary risk of genetic diseases. Expenses involved for egg or sperm donation or surrogacy all vary from facility to facility. Here is a general breakdown of estimated costs involved for egg donation:

Donors fee- $2,000-$5,000

Donors fertility medications- $3,000

Donors cycle fees (ultrasounds, labs, pain meds, etc)- $2,500

Donors egg retrieval procedure (Transfer, lab costs) - $3,000

Facility fee - $1,500

Recipient cycle costs (ultrasounds, meds, labs, cycle management, sperm prep, follow up care, etc) - $12,000

Initial embryo freezing - $750

- Adoption is an excellent option; however it is not for everyone. Some welcome the opportunity to bring a child who has no one into their family and home. Others struggle with the thought of it still being an adopted child. They wonder if they will ever be able to love a child they are not biologically linked to as much as they would love their own child. If this is the route you decide upon, there are questions you need to think about.

Do you want a boy or a girl?

What age do you prefer?

Are you interested in a particular race?

Will a disability deter you?

Do you want an open or closed adoption?

Are you going to change the name of the child?

Once you're ready and know what you want, the next step is finding the right agency. You can find them in the yellow pages, online and word of mouth. Compile a list of the ones you are most interested in to talking to. When you call them, here is a list of questions to inquire about:

What is the availability of the age group you're interested in?

What are the adoption requirements?

Is there a waiting list?

What is the adoption policy for open or closed adoptions?

What are the procedures for the home visit and placement?

What are the fees involved?

Typically adopting a child that has special needs or one that is older from your state social services department has financial benefits. Usually the amount you would have to pay out of pocket is very small, if anything at all. Private adoptions on the other hand can be very costly. Both domestic and international adoptions can bring a price tag anywhere from $15,000-$40,000. Most families who adopt are eligible for a tax credit from the federal government.

Our friends and family certainly mean well as they divulge every detail on the tricks that got them pregnant. What happens when you have tried them all and then some and you still aren't pregnant? What do you do when it is time to move on? How can you put all your hopes and dreams of being a mother to rest?

The truth is, my dear cyster, it will never be easy to make the decision of calling it a day. Our hearts, arms and wombs will always long to have a bundle of joy there. There are many reasons why it may be absolutely necessary to be done though. It's possible you have exhausted all your finances. Let's face it, nothing about infertility is cheap. Not only that, it takes a serious toll on you mentally and physically. How many IVF cycles can one person go through only to come out unsuccessful?

Tip:

Write a letter to your "child." Open your heart to them; share your hopes that you had for them and as a family. Tell them goodbye. It's up to you what you decide to do with the letter. Maybe release it in a balloon, bury it in a keepsake box, store it in a bible, picture frame, journal, etc.

CHAPTER 11- CONTRACEPTION OPTIONS

Maybe you aren't trying to get pregnant, if fact maybe you're trying to prevent it. This is the chapter for you. We will discuss various birth control options and what they entail.

Having children is not at the top of everyone's agenda. Thankfully there are many contraceptive options available to prevent pregnancy. When considering birth control, here are few questions to help determine which option is best for you and your current situation:

- How affordable is it
- Will it protect me from STI's
- Is it effective
- Is it safe
- How easy is it to use
- Is it reversible

FUN FACT

<u>Did you know in 1916 Margaret Sanger opened the world's first birth control clinic. This was during a time that distributing information about birth control was illegal.</u>

Contraceptive options

~ Male Condom: Sheath that covers the penis. They are inexpensive and very easy to get. They are not complicated to use and do not alter a woman's hormone levels.
~ Female condom: also called a vaginal pouch. This is a long sheath that has flexible rings on both ends. One end is inserted into your vagina just how you would use a diaphragm.

They can be put in a few hours before you have sex. Like male condoms, they do not alter female hormone levels. FDA approved these in 1993.

~ Diaphragm: This is a reusable round cup like device with flexible rings on both ends. It covers the cervix which prevents sperm from getting into the uterus. Using a diaphragm with spermicide will increase its effectiveness.

~ Cervical cap: very similar to a diaphragm except it is shaped more like a cap as the name implies. It is also much smaller than a diaphragm. A cervical cap is held in its place by a suction effect and fits right over the cervix.

Male and female condoms can be purchased over the counter however diaphragms and cervical caps require a prescription and a pelvic exam to have it fitted to find the right size for you. Neither device interferes with hormone levels. They typically can't be felt by you or your partner during sex.

All four options are considered barrier contraceptives. Your "fertility" does not change with use. This means immediately after your last use it is possible to get pregnant if you do not use another one. The effectiveness on all four options is increased when you use a spermicidal cream with them. A spermicide is a chemical that does not hurt us but stops the sperm from being able to join the egg. They come in many forms; cream, jelly and foam. These are fairly inexpensive and sold over the counter, typically in close proximity to the condoms. Spermicides do not affect hormone levels.

FUN FACT

<u>Around 3,000 BC, they used condoms made from animal intestines and fish bladders. Years later they began making them from linen or silk.</u>

~ Intrauterine Device (IUD): Flexible piece of plastic with a string attached to the bottom. The IUD fits inside of the uterus with the attached string hanging through the opening of the cervix. IUD's are available with prescription only and are removed by your doctor. They typically stay in for a few years and once removed your fertility should return to normal almost immediately. If needed, it can be removed sooner by a simple visit to your doctor. IUD's are not felt by you or your partner during sex. There are two different kinds of IUD's. One kind is the paraGard T380A. This is T shaped, and partially covered by copper. Usually works for 10 years. The second type is Progestasert. This is T shaped as well and contains progestin which is released over a year period. A few examples of IUD's are Mirena and Nuvaring.

~ Implantable contraceptives: Implanon is a small rod, smaller than a toothpick; approximately 2mm by 4cm. It is inserted with a local anesthetic on the underside of your non dominant upper arm, just under the skin. A progestin called Etonogestrel is released by it. The procedure usually takes 15-20 minutes and you don't need stitches after. It should go into effect within a day or so after insertion and will work for up to 3 years. In order to prevent pregnancy, a new implant will need to be inserted immediately after removal. Some of the most common side effects are changes in menstrual cycles like a heavier flow, spotting, cessation of periods, and changes in cycle length. Some of the less common side effects are headaches, weight gain, acne, nausea, nervousness and breast tenderness.

~ Shot: also known as injections of Depotmedroxyprogesterone Acetate or DMPA for short. This is injected into the muscle on your arm or butt. It's commonly referred to as Depo-Provera. This is able to prevent pregnancy for 12-14 weeks by stopping your ovaries from releasing any eggs. It offers no protection from sexually transmitted infections. The most common side effect of Depo- Provera is cessation of periods. Some of the less common side effects are headaches, nervousness, depression, breast tenderness, and weight gain.

~ Tubal Ligation: Also known as "having your tubes tied". It is done by blocking, tying or cutting the fallopian tubes. If you decide you want children after the procedure, you will need to undergo surgery.

Birth control pill:

Your fertility should return somewhere up to 2 months after the pill is stopped.

If you have any of the following conditions, the pill should not be taken:

o Breast cancer   Uterine cancer   Stroke
o Undiagnosed vaginal bleeding   Active Liver Disease   Heart Disease
o History of leg or chest clots

A few examples of the birth control pill are: Marvelon, Yasmin, Ocella, and Yaz.

The pill carries some excellent benefits:

- Fewer tubal pregnancies
- Reduced acne

- Less excess body hair
- Reduced risk of cancer of the ovary and uterus
- 50% less pelvic infection
- Less likelihood of endometriosis
- 50%-80% fewer ovarian cysts
- Lighter, predictable and less painful periods
- Less premenstrual tension and period pain
- No menopausal symptoms while on it
- Safe and reversible pregnancy prevention

FUN FACT

In 1873 the Comstock Act passed allowing the USPS to confiscate any birth control items sold via the postal service. This act also prohibited advertising and distributing information on birth control.

Some of the most common side effects of the birth control pill usually happen within the first three months of use. They are:

- Lighter menstrual flow
- Spotting
- Changes in period length
- Cessation of periods
- Abdominal cramping
- Bloating
- Fatigue
- Dizziness
- Nausea
- Vomiting
- Breast tenderness or swelling

If the birth control pill is your contraceptive of choice, be aware that certain medications can interfere with it.

The following medications are **less effective** while on the birth control pill.

- ✧ Analgesics
  -Acetaminophen (Pamprin, Tylenol, Paracetamol, Aspirin free Excedrin)

- ✧ Anticoagulants
  -Warfarin (Coumadin, Panwarfin)
- ✧ Antihypertensives
  -Methyldopa (Aldoclor, Aldomet)
- ✧ Hypoglycemics
  -Diabinese
  -Orinase
  -Tolbutamide
  -Tolinase

Fertility Abbreviations

AF Aunt Flow

AI Artificial Insemination

AID Artificial Insemination from Donor

AIH Artificial Insemination from Husband

ANS Autonomic Nervous System

AO Anovulation

ART Assisted Reproductive Technology

ASRM American Society for Reproductive Medicine

BBT Basal Body Temperature

BCE Before The Common Era

BCP Birth Control Pills

BD Baby Dance (Intercourse)

BFN Big Fat Negative (Pregnancy Test)

BFP Big Fat Positive (Pregnancy Test)

BG Blood Glucose

BTB Break Through Bleeding

BW, b/w Bloodwork

C# Cycle Number

CBC Complete Blood Count

CD Cycle Day

CDC Centers for Disease Control and Prevention

CE Common Era

CF Cervical Fluid

CM Cervical Mucus

COH Controlled Ovarian Hyperstimulation

CP Cervical Position

D&C Dilation and Curettage

D&E Dilation and Evacuation

DE Donor Egg(s)

DHEAS Dehydroepiandrosterone Sulfate

DI Donor Insemination

DOR Diminished Ovarian Reserve

DPO Days Post Ovulation

DPR Days Post Retrieval

DPT Days Post Transfer

DRI Dietary Reference Intake

Dx Diagnosis

E2 Estradiol (Estrogen)

EDC Estimated Date of Conception

EDD Estimated Due Date

EPT Early Pregnancy Test

ERT Estrogen Replacement Therapy

ET Embryo Transfer

EW Egg White

EWCF Egg White Cervical Fluid

EXCM Egg White Cervical Mucus

FBG Fasting Blood Glucose

FDA Food and Drug Administration

FET Frozen Embryo Transfer

FHR Fetal Heart Rate

FMU First Morning Urine

FSH Follicle Stimulating Hormone

GD Gestational Diabetes

GnRH Gonadotropin Releasing Hormone

GP General Practitioner

GTT Glucose Tolerance Test

HbA1C Glycosylated Hemoglobin

HCG Human Chorionic Gonadotropin

HCP Health Care Practitioner

HPT Home Pregnancy Test

HRT Hormone Replacement Therapy

HSC Hysteroscopy

HSG Hysterosalpingogram

ICI Intra Cervical Insemination

IF Infertility

IGTT Insulin and Glucose Tolerance Test

IM Intra Muscular (Injection)

IR Insulin Resistant

IUD Intra Uterine Device

IUI Intra Uterine Insemination

IVF In Vitro Fertilization

LEEP Loop Electrosurgical Excision Procedure

LH Luteinizing Hormone

LMP Last Menstrual Period

LOD Laparoscopic Ovarian Drilling

LP Luteal Phase

LPD Luteal Phase Defect

LSP Low Sperm Count

MAOI Monoamine Oxidase Inhibitor

MC, m/c Miscarriage

NP Nurse Practitioner

O, OV Ovulation

OB Obstetrician

OB/GYN Obstetrician/ Gynecologist

OC Oral Contraceptive

OCP Oral Contraceptive Pill

OD Ovulatory Dysfunction

OHSS Ovarian Hyperstimulation Syndrome

OI Ovulation Induction

OPK Ovulation Predictor Kit

OPT Ovulation Predictor Test

OTC Over The Counter

P4 Progesterone

PA Physician's Assistant

PCAO Poly Cystic Appearing Ovaries

PCO Poly Cystic Ovaries

PCOD Poly Cystic Ovarian Disease

PCOS Poly Cystic Ovarian Syndrome

PCP Primary Care Physician

PG Pregnant/ Pregnancy

PI Primary Infertility

PID Pelvic Inflammatory Disease

PMS Premenstrual Syndrome

POF Premature Ovarian Failure

RDA Recommended Dietary Allowance

RE Reproductive Endocrinologist

RPL Recurrent Pregnancy Loss

RSA Recurrent Spontaneous Abortion

Rx Prescription

S/B Still Birth

SA Semen Analysis

SC Subcutaneous (injection)

SERM Selective Estrogen Receptor Modulator

SHBG Sex Hormone Binding Globulin

SI Secondary Infertility

SSRI Selective Serotonin Reuptake Inhibitor

T4 Thyroxine

TL Tubal Ligation

TR Tubal Reversal

TSH Thyroid Stimulating Hormone

TTC Trying To Conceive

TWW, 2WW Two Week Wait

Tx Treatment

US, u/s Ultrasound

UTI Urinary Tract Infection

WBC White Blood Cells

WNL Within Normal Limits

Glossary

Abortion- Termination of pregnancy

Adrenal Gland- Endocrine gland above each kidney that secretes the hormones adrenaline, androgen, estrogen and progesterone

Amenorrhea- Prolonged absence of menstruation

Androgens- Male sex hormones

Anovulation- Absence of ovulation

Anovulatory Cycle- Cycle where ovulation doesn't occur

Aphrodisiac- Substance used to heighten sexual desire

Artificial Insemination- Procedure where syringe is used to insert sperm just in or outside of the cervix

Basal Body Temperature- Body temperature taken in the early morning before rising

Blighted Ovum- Pregnancy where no fetus developed in pregnancy sac

Carb- Sugars and starches

Cervical Mucus- Produced by cervical canal

Cervix- Lower portion of uterus that projects into the vagina

Chi- Chinese term for an energy force that flows through your body

Chronic- Long term

Colposcopy- Procedure used to examine vagina and cervix under magnification through colposcope

Conceive- To become pregnant

Condom- Sheath of thin rubber worn over penis to prevent pregnancy

Contraception- Prevention of pregnancy by artificial means

Corpus Luteum- Yellow gland formed by ruptured follicle after ovulation. If fertilization doesn't occur, it degenerates within 12-16 days

Corpus Luteum Cyst- Formed when the corpus luteum fails to shrink after ovulation

Cortisol- Stress hormone

Depo provera- Birth control injection

DHEAS- Testosterone hormone

Diaphragm- Birth control cap like device coated with spermicide placed inside vagina to block cervix

Dysmenorrhea- Painful menstruation

Dyspareunia- Painful or difficult intercourse

Early Ovulation- Release of an egg earlier in cycle than usual or anticipated

Ectopic Pregnancy- Implantation and development of fertilized ovum outside of the uterus

Embryo- Earliest stage of baby development

Endocrine System- System of glands in the body that releases hormones into the bloodstream

Endocrinologist- Physician who specializes in function of hormones

Endometrial Biopsy- Removal of small part of uterine lining to determine if it is developing appropriately

Endometrium- Lining of the uterus, shed during menstruation

Estradiol- Hormone produced by ovary. It helps follicles grow and prepares uterine lining for pregnancy

Estrogen- Group of hormones produced by the ovaries

Ferning Test- Characteristic pattern produced by fertile cervical fluid when dried on a glass slide

Fertile Phase- The cycle days when pregnancy may occur

Fertility- Ability to produce offspring

Fertility Drugs- Drugs used to stimulate ovulation

Fertilization- Fusion of sperm with an egg

Follicle- Fluid filled saw with maturing egg

Follicular Cyst- Formed when a follicle has grown in preparation for ovulation but fails to rupture and release the egg

Follicular Fluid- Fluid inside of the follicle

Functional Cyst- A cyst that arises from normal ovarian functions during menstrual cycle

FSH- Hormone produced by the pituitary gland that stimulates ovaries to produce mature ova and estrogen

General Anesthesia- Causing temporary loss of consciousness and inability to feel pain by use of inhaled gasses or injected anesthetics

Glucose Load- Eating

Gluten- Protein found in wheat

GnRH- Chemical substance produced by hypothalamus in brain. It stimulates pituitary gland to produce and release FSH and LH

Gonadotropins- Hormone produced by the pituitary gland that regulates maturation of egg. Most important gonadotropins are FSH and LH

Guaifenesin- Expectorant taken to increase fluidity of cervical fluid

Gynecologist- Doctor who specializes in woman's reproductive health

HCG- Pregnancy hormone produced by the developing embryo when implanted in uterine lining

Hormone- Chemical substances produced in one organ and carried to another to work

HRT- Use of manufactured hormones to replace diminished supply

HSG- Xray taken after injected with dye through the cervix to see the inside of the uterus and tubes to check for blockages or scarring

Hydrosalpinx- Blocked fluid filled fallopian tube

Hypermenorrhea- Heavy bleeding

Hypomenorrhea- Light flow or spotting

Hypothalamus- Part of the brain that controls the pituitary gland

Hysterectomy- Surgical removal of uterus

Hysteroscopy- Exploratory surgery to view uterus

Idiopathic Infertility- Unknown cause of infertility

Infertile Phase- A time when pregnancy cannot occur

Infertility- Inability to conceive or maintain a pregnancy

Intra Muscular- Injection deep into the muscle of the buttocks with a 1 ½ inch needle

IUD- Device place in cavity of uterus to prevent pregnancy

IUI- Procedure where catheter is used to insert sperm through cervix to uterus

IVF- A procedure where eggs are fertilized in a petri dish and then place into the uterus days later

LEEP- Surgery to remove thin piece of cervical tissue to diagnosis abnormalities or remove precancerous or cancerous tissue

LH- Hormone from pituitary gland that is released in a surge to start ovulation and development of corpus luteum

Local Anesthesia- Temporary prevention of pain in a limited and usually superficial area of the body by injecting medication

Low tech Tx- Treatment that doesn't require egg retrieval and manipulation

Luteal Phase- Phase of cycle from ovulation to onset of next period

Menarche- Very first menstrual cycle

Metabolic Resistance- Condition when a person's BMR is so low they have a difficult time losing weight

Norplant- Set of 6 plastic tubes implanted under the forearm of a woman's skin that releases controlled doses of birth control over five years

Oligomenorrhea- Periods that occur more than 35 days apart

Oophorectomy- Ovary removal

Ova- Egg cells (plural)

Ovarian Diathermy- Keyhole surgery to burn cysts off of ovaries in an effort to restore ovulation

Ovulation- Release of maturing egg from follicle

Polymenorrhea- Frequent bleeding usually due to anovulation

Prophylactic- Preventative

Reproductive Endocrinologist- Doctor who specializes in reproductive hormones

Rhizome- Underground stems

Subcutaneous- Injection given just under the skin, with a ¼ inch needle Usually in upper thigh or abdominal area

Ultrasound-

Abdominal: Uses sound waves to create an image similar to a radar. Requires the sound beams to pass through your skin, fat, muscles and organs to see your ovary.

Vaginal: Small probe around an inch wide. It is covered by a sheath similar to a condom and coated with a gel for lubrication

Xeno Oestrogen- Any oestrogen like substance, not of plant origin that has been introduced into the body

17 Hydroxyprogesterone- Hormone made by both ovaries and adrenal glands

Measurements

Pg/mL Picograms per milliliter

Ng/mL Nanograms per milliliter

MIU/mL One million international units per milliliter

C, c Cup

G Gram

Gr Grain

Kg Kilogram

L, l Liter

Lb Pound

Mg Milligram

Mcg Microgram

ML Milliliter

Oz Ounce

Pt Pint

T, Tsp Teaspoon

Tbl, tbsp Tablespoon

IU International Unit

RE Retinol Equivalent

mmHg Millimeters of mercury

MM millimeters

MMOL/L Millimoles per litre

Ng/ml Nanograms per milliliter

Nmol/l nanomoles per litre

u/l units per litre

umol/l micromoles per litre

USP Unit   United States Pharmacopeia

MDR   Minimum Daily Requirement

AMDR   Adult Minimum Daily Requirement

Credentials

Acupuncture-

C.A Certified Acupuncturist

Dipl. Ac Diplomat of Acupuncture

L.Ac/ Lic. Ac Licensed Acupuncturist

M.Ac Master of Acupuncture

R.Ac Registered Acupuncturist

N.C.C.A National Commission for Certification of Acupuncturists

NCCAOM National Certification Commission provides certification for Acupuncture and Oriental Medicine

AAMA Practitioner is a member of the American Academy of Medical Acupuncturists. It is only open to medical doctors and doctors of osteopathy.

Acupressure-

AOBTA American Organization for Body Work Therapies of Asia

DiplABT Diplomat in Asian Body Work Therapy

NCBTMB National Certified Board for Therapeutic Massage and Body Work

Aromatherapy-

NAHA National Association for Holistic Aromatherapy

RA Registered Aromatherapist

Ayurveda-

B.A.M.S Bachelor of Ayurveda Medical Studies

DAMS Doctor of Ayurvedic Medicine and Surgery

Chiropractic-

D.C Doctor of Chiropractic

Homeopathy-

C.C.H Certified in Classical Homeopathy

D.H Diplomat in Homeopathy

DHANP Diplomat of Homeopathic Academy of Naturopathic Physicians

L.H.P Licensed Homeopathic Physician

M.D (H.) Doctor of Homeopathic Medicine

Hypnotherapy-

C.H Certified Hypnotherapist

Naturopathy-

N.D Doctor of Naturopathic Medicine

Psychiatrist-

M.D Medical Doctor

Massage-

C.M.P/C.M.T Certified Massage Practitioner/ Therapist

L.M.P/L.M.T Licensed Massage Practitioner/ Therapist

Nutritional Counseling-

C.N.C Certified Nutritional Consultant

L.D Licensed Dietitian

R.D Registered Dietitian

D.T Dietetic Technician

Mental Health Counselor-

M.A Master of Arts

M.Ed Master of Education

Psychologist-

Ed.D Doctor of Education

M.A Master of Arts

Ph.D Doctor of Philosophy

Psy.D Doctor of Psychology

Social Worker-

A.C.S.W Academy of Certified Social Workers

B.C.D Board Certified Diplomat in Clinical Social Work

C.S.W Certified Social Work

D.S.W Doctor of Social Work

L.C.S.W Licensed Clinical Social Worker

L.I.C.S.W Licensed Independent Clinical Social Worker

M.S.W Master of Social Work

PhD Doctor of Philosophy

Reiki-

R.M Reiki Master

Traditional Chinese Medicine-

D.O.M/O.M.D Doctor of Oriental Medicine

M.O.M Master of Oriental Medicine

Dip.Phyto Diplomate of Phytotherapy

RH Registered Herbalist

General-

R.N Registered Nurse

R.Ph Registered Pharmacist

P.A Physician's Assistant

M.B Bachelor of Medicine

C.M.A Certified Medical Assistant

L.P.N Licensed Practical Nurse

C.N.M Certified Nurse Midwife

D.Div Doctor of Divinity

DDS Doctor of Dental Surgery

D.I.B.A.K Diplomat of the International Board of Applied Kinesiology

Dipl. C.H Diplomat of Chinese Herbology

D.M.D Doctor of Dental Medicine

M. Div Master of Divinity

M.H Master Herbalist

M.S.N Master of Science in Nursing

P.T Physical Therapist

Degrees-

B.M Bachelor of Medicine

B.M.T Bachelor of Medical Technology

B.N. Bachelor of Nursing

B.S.N Bachelor of Science in Nursing

C.A.E Certified Association Executive

C.C.C-A Certificate of Clinical Competence Audiology

D.Ed Department of Education

M.A Master of Arts

M.O.H Master of Occupational Health

M.P.H Master of Public Health

M.S Master of Science

Titles in organizations

F.A.A.P Fellow, American Academy of Pediatrics

F.A.A.O.S Fellow, American Academy of Orthopedic Surgeons

F.A.A.D Fellow, American Academy of Dermatology

F.A.A.F.P Fellow, American Academy of Family Physicians

F.A.C.C Fellow, American College of Cardiology

F.A.C.E Fellow, American College of Endocrinology

F.A.C.O.G Fellow, American College of Obstetricians and Gynecologists

F.A.C.P Fellow, American College of Physicians

F.A.C.S Fellow, American College of Surgeons

F.C.C.P Fellow, American College of Chest Physicians

F.I.C.C Fellow, International College of Chiropractors

F.N.A.A.O.M Fellow, National Academy of Acupuncture & Oriental Medicine

M.A.C.P Master, American College of Physicians

Resources

*National Center for Complementary and Alternative Medicine

NCCAM Clearinghouse

PO Box 7923

Gaithersburg, MD 20898

888-644-6226

http://www.nccam.nih.gov

*American Fertility Association

666 Fifth Avenue Suite 278

New York, NY 10103

888-917-3777

http://www.theafa.org

*American Board of Obstetrics and Gynecology

2915 Vine Street

Dallas, Tx 75204

214-871-1614

http://www.abog.org

*Polycystic Ovarian Syndrome Association

PO Box 3403

Englewood, CO 80111

877-775-7267

http://www.pcossupport.org

*The Ayurvedic Institute

11311 Menaul NE

Albuquerque, NM 87112

505-291-9698

http://www.ayurveda.com

*American Sleep Apnea Association

Washington, DC 20005

202-293-3650

http://www.sleepapnea.org

*American Association of Oriental Medicine

433 Front Street

Catasauqua, PA 18032

610-433-2448

*American Academy of Medical Acupuncture

323-937-5514

http://www.medicalacupuncture.org

*The National Association for Holistic Aromatherapy

4509 Interlake Avenue North #233

Seattle, WA 98103

888-ASK-NAHA

http://www.naha.gov

*American Chiropractic Association

1701 Claredon Boulevard

Arlington, VA 22209

703-276-8800

http://www.amerchiro.org

*National Institutes of Health (NCCAM)

9000 Rockville Pike

Bethesda, MD 20892

http://www.nccam.nih.gov

*American Alliance of Aromatherapy

PO Box 750428

Petaluma, CA 94975

707-778-6762

*American Aromatherapy Association

PO Box 3679

South Pasadena, CA 91031

818-457-1742

*Academy for Guided Imagery

PO Box 2070

Mill Valley, CA 94942

800-726-2070

*The American Institute of Hypnotherapy

1805 East Garryn Avenue Suite 100

Santa Ana, CA 92705

714-261-6400

*American Massage Therapy Association (AMTA)

820 Davis Street Suite 100

Evanston, IL 60201

847-864-0123

*Insight Meditation Society

1230 Pleasant Street

Barre, MA 01005

508-355-4378

*Homeopathic Educational Services

2124 Kittredge Street

Berkeley, CA 94704

510-649-0294

http://www.homeopathic.com

*The Infertility Network

160 Pikering Street

Toronto, CA

http://www.infertilitynetwork.org

*RESOLVE, Inc

7910 Woodmont Avenue Suite 1350

Bethesda, MD 20814

301-652-8585

http://www.resolve.org

*American Heart Association

7272 Greenville Avenue

Dallas, TX 75231

800-242-8721

http://www.americanheart.org

*National Center for Complementary and Alternative Medicine (NCCAM)

888-644-6226

http://www.nccam.nih.gov

*Fertility Lifelines

866-LETS-TRY (538-7879)

http://www.fertilitylifelines.com

*Center for Surrogate Parenting

15821 Ventura Boulevard, Suite 675

Encino, CA 91436

818-788-8288

http://www.creatingfamilies.com

*Anxiety Disorders Association of America

8730 Georgia Ave, Suite 600

Silver Spring, MD 20910

240-485-1001

http://www.adaa.org

*American Psychiatric Association

1000 Wilson Blvd, Suite 1825

Arlington, VA 22209

703-907-7300

http:://www.psych.org

*Mental Health America

2000 N. Beauregard St. 6th Floor

Alexandria, VA 22311

http://www.nmha.org

*American Society of Hypertension

148 Madison Ave, 5th floor

New York, NY 10016

212-696-9099

http://www.ash-us.org

*American Heart Association

7272 Greenville Ave

Dallas, TX 75231

800-242-8721

http://www.americanheart.org

*National Sleep Foundation

1522 K Street NW, Suite 500

Washington, DC 20005

202-347-3471

http://www.sleepfoundation.org

*American Association of Clinical Endocrinologists

245 Riverside Ave, Suite 200

Jacksonville, FL 32202

904-353-7878

http://www.aace.com

*Endocrine Society

8401 Connecticut Ave, Suite 900

Chevy Chase, MD 20815

301-941-0200

http://www.endo-society.org

*American Sleep Apnea Association

1424 K Street NW, Suite 302

Washington, DC 20005

202-293-3650

http://www.sleepapnea.org

*American Academy of Dermatology

PO Box 4014

Schaumburg, IL 60618

866-503-7546

http://www.aad.org

*American Society for Reproductive Medicine

1209 Montgomery Highway

Birmingham, AL 35216

205-978-5000

http://www.asrm.org

*National Heart, Lung & Blood Institute Information Center

PO Box 30105

Bethesda, MD 20824

301-592-8573

http://www.nhlbi.nih.gov

*National Women's Health Resource Center

157 Broad St. Suite 315

Red Bank, NJ 07701

877-986-9472

http://www.healthywomen.org

*Ferre Institute, Inc

124 Front Street

Binghamton, NY 13905

607-724-4308

http://www.ferre.org

*Food and Drug Administration

5600 Fishers Lane

Rockville, MD 20857

888-INFO-FDA

http://www.FDA.gov

*American Dietetic Association

120 S. Riverside Plaza, Suite 2000

Chicago, IL 60606

800-877-1600

http://www.eatright.org

Books:

*Minerals, Supplements and Vitamins, The essential guide by H. Winter Griffith, M.D

*The Insulin Resistance diet by Cheryle R. Hart, M.D and Mary Kay Grossman R.D

*The Low GI Diet Revolution by Dr. Jennie Brand-Miller and Kaye Foster Powell

Websites:

http://www.reflexology.org

http://www.sharedjourney.com

http://www.inciid.org

http://www.fertilethoughts.com

http://www.massagetherapy101.com

http://massagetherapy.com

http://www.olen.com/food (Fast food finder)

http://www.nal.usda.gov/fnic/foodcomp/ (Nutrient Data Laboratory)

http://www.acebabes.co.uk (For families who conceived through assisted conception)

http://www.herbalgram.org American Botanical Council

http://www.ahpa.org American Herbal Products Association

http://www.NCCAOM.org

http://www.aobta.org American Organization for Bodywork Therapies of Asia

http://www.aaaomonline.org American Association of Acupuncture and Oriental Medicine

http://www.acupuncture.com

http://www.aromatherapycouncil.org Aromatherapy Registration Council

http://www.naha.org National Association for Holistic Aromatherapy

http://www.ayurveda.com Ayurvedic Institute

http://www.Amerchiro.org American Chiropractic Association (ACA)

http://www.flowersociety.org Flower Essence Society (FES)

http://www.holisticmedicine.org American Holistic Medicine Association (AHMA)

http://www.homeopathic.org National Center for Homeopath

http://www.asch.net American Society of Clinical Hypnosis

http://www.ngh.net National Guild of Hypnotists, Inc

http://www.smokefree.gov

http://www.naturopathic.org American Association of Naturopath Physicians

http://www.aanc.net American Association of Nutritional Consultants

http://www.reflexology-usa.net International Institute of Reflexology

http://www.IAYT.org International Association of Yoga Therapists (IAYT)

http://www.altmedicine.net Alternative Medicine Directory

http://www.medicalacupuncture.org American Association of Medical Acupuncture

Poison Control 800-222-1222

References

Chapter 1

1. Hanson AE. Hippocrates: Diseases of women 1. Signs (chic) 1975; 1:567-84 [Pubmed]
2. Temkin O. Soranus' Gynecology. The John Hopkins University Press; Baltimore: 1991
3. Rosner F, Munter S. The Medical Aphorism of Moses Maimonides, Vol. II. Yeshiva University Press; New York: 1971
4. Wild RA, Long term health consequences of PCOS Human Reproductive Update, 2008; 8:231-241
5. www.pcosinstitute.com
6. www.mcdowellhouse.com/history/ephraim-mcdowell

Chapter 2

1. Knochenhaur ES, Key TJ, Kahsar Miller M, Waggoner W, Boots LR, Azziz R. Prevalence of the Polycystic Ovary Syndrome in unselected black and white women of the southeastern United States: A prospective study. J Clin Endocrinol Metab. 1998;83:3078-82
2. http://www.nature.com/ijo/journal/v26/n7/full/0801994a.html International Journel of Obesity

3. vhttp://www.aace.com/files/american-college-of-endocrinology-position-statement-on-the-insulin-resistance-syndrome.pdf

4. http://www.reproductivefacts.org

Chapter 10
1. http://www.ivf-worldwide.com/ivf-history.html